CONTENTS.

"The choice and measure of the materials of which our Body is composed,—and what we take daily by Pounds,—is at least of as much importance as what we take seldom, and only by *Grains* and *Spoonsful*."—Dr. Arbuthnot on *Aliment,* pref. p. iii.

The Editor of the following pages had originally an extremely Delicate Constitution;—and at an early period devoted himself to the study of Physic, with the hope—of learning how to make the most of his small stock of Health.

The System he adopted, succeeded, and he is arrived at his forty-third year, in tolerable good Health; and this without any uncomfortable abstinence:— his maxim has ever been, *"dum Vivimus, Vivamus."*

He does not mean the Aguish existence of the votary of Fashion—whose Body is burning from voluptuous intemperance to-day, and freezing in miserable collapse to-morrow—not extravagantly consuming in a Day, the animal spirits which Nature intended for the animation of a Week—but keeping the expense of the machinery of Life within the income of Health, —which the Constitution can regularly and comfortably supply.

This is the grand "arcanum duplicatum" for "Living all the days of your Life."

The Art of Invigorating the Health, and improving the Strength of Man, has hitherto only been considered for the purpose of training[1] him for Athletic Exercises—but I have often thought that a similar plan might be adopted with considerable advantage, to animate and strengthen enfeebled Constitutions—prevent Gout—reduce Corpulency—cure Nervous and Chronic Weakness—Hypochondriac and Bilious Disorders, &c.—*to*

increase the Enjoyment, and prolong the duration of Feeble Life—for which *Medicine*, unassisted by DIET AND REGIMEN,—affords but very trifling and temporary help.

The universal desire of repairing, perfecting, and prolonging Life, has induced many ingenious men to try innumerable experiments on almost all the products of the Animal, Vegetable, and Mineral kingdoms, with the hope of discovering Agents, that will not merely increase or diminish the force or frequency of the Pulse; but with an ardour as romantic as the search after the Philosopher's Stone, they have vainly hoped, that *Panaceas* might be found possessing the power of curing "all the evils that flesh is heir to."

This is evident enough to all who have examined the early Pharmacopœias, which are full of heterogeneous compounds, the inventions of interested, and the imaginations of ignorant men.

The liberal and enlightened Physicians of the last and present century have gradually expunged most of these, and made the science of Medicine sufficiently intelligible to those whose business it is to learn it—if Medicine be entirely divested of its Mystery, its power over the Mind, which in most cases forms its main strength, will no longer exist.

It was a favourite remark of the celebrated Dr. John Brown[2], that "if a student in Physic employed seven years in storing his memory with the accepted, but,—unfortunately, in nine cases out of ten,—imaginary powers of Medicine, he would, if he did not possess very extraordinary sagacity, lose a much longer time in discovering the multiform delusions his medical oracles had imposed upon him—before he ascertains that, with the exception of *Mercury* for the Lues,—*Bark* for Intermittents,—and *Sulphur* for Psora—the *Materia Medica* does not furnish many Specifics—and may be almost reduced to Evacuants and Stimuli:"—However, these, skilfully administered, afford all the assistance to Nature, that can be obtained from Art!

Let not the uninitiated in Medical Mysteries imagine for a moment, that the Editor desires to depreciate their Importance—but observe once for all—that he has only one reason for writing this Book—which is, to warn you against the ordinary causes of Disorder—and to teach you the easiest and most salutary method of preventing or subduing it, and of recovering and preserving Health and Strength, when, in spite of all your prudence, you are overtaken by sickness, and have no Medical Friend ready to defend you.

Experience has so long proved the actual importance of TRAINING—that Pugilists will not willingly engage without such preparation.

The principal rules for which are,—to go to Bed early—to Rise early—to take as much *Exercise* as you can in the open air, without fatigue—to *Eat and Drink* moderately of plain nourishing Food—and especially,—to keep *the Mind* diverted[3], and in as easy and cheerful a state as possible.

Somewhat such a system is followed at the fashionable watering places—and great would be the improvement of Health that would result from it,—if it was not continually counteracted, by visits to the Ball Room[4] and the Card Table.

A residence in the Country will avail little, if you carry with you there, the irregular habits, and late hours of fashionable Life.

Do not expect much benefit from mere change of *Air*—the purest breezes of the country will produce very little effect, unless accompanied by plenty of regular *Exercise*[5]—*Temperance*—and, above all, *Tranquillity of Mind.*— See *Obs. on* "AIR" and "EXERCISE."

The following is a brief sketch of the usual METHOD OF TRAINING PERSONS FOR ATHLETIC EXERCISES.

The Alimentary Canal[6] is cleansed by an Emetic, and then two or three Purgatives.—See *Index.*

They are directed to eat Beef and Mutton[7]—rather *under*, than *over*-done, and without either Seasoning or Sauce—*Broils*, (No. 94), are preferred to either *Roasts* (No. 19), or *Boils*—and stale Bread or Biscuit.

Neither Veal—Lamb—Pork—Fish—Milk—Butter—Cheese—Puddings—Pastry—or Vegetables, are allowed.

Beef and Mutton only (fresh, not salted) are ordered;—but we believe this restriction is seldom entirely submitted to.

Nothing tends more to renovate the Constitution, than a temporary retirement to the Country.

The necessity of breathing a pure Air, and the strictest Temperance, are uniformly and absolutely insisted upon by all Trainers;—the striking advantages resulting therefrom, we have heard as universally acknowledged by those who have been trained.

Mild Home-brewed Ale is recommended for Drink—about three pints per day—taken with Breakfast and Dinner, and a little at Supper—not in large draughts—but by mouthfuls, alternately with your food.

Stale Beer often disturbs delicate Bowels—if your Palate warns you that Malt Liquor is inclined to be hard, neutralize it with a little *Carbonate of Potash*;—that good sound Beer, which is neither nauseous from its newness, nor noxious from its staleness, is in unison with the animating diet of Animal Food, which we are recommending as the most effective antidote to debility, &c. experience has sufficiently proved.—There can be no doubt, that the combination of the tonic power of the Hop, and the nourishment of the Malt, is much more invigorating than any simple vinous spirit,—but the difficulty of obtaining it good, ready brewed—and the trouble of Brewing is so great—that happy are those who are contented with Good Toast and Water (No. 463*), as a diluent to solid food—and a few glasses of wine as a finishing "*Bonne Bouche.*"

Those who do not like Beer—are allowed Wine and Water—Red wine is preferred to White, and *not more* than half a pint, (*i. e.* eight ounces), or four common sized wine glasses, after Dinner—none after Supper—nor any Spirits, however diluted.

Eight hours' *Sleep* are necessary—but this is generally left to the previous habits of the Person; those who take active Exercise, require adequate Rest.

BREAKFAST[8] upon meat at eight o'clock—DINNER at two—SUPPER is not advised, but they may have a little bit of cold meat about eight o'clock, and take a walk after, between it and ten, when they go to Bed.

The Time requisite to screw a Man up to his fullest Strength, depends upon his previous habits and Age. In the Vigour of Life, between 20 and 35, a Month or two is generally sufficient:—more or less, according as he is older, and as his previous Habits have been in opposition to the above system.

By this mode of proceeding for two or three months—the Constitution of the human frame is greatly improved, and the Courage proportionately increased,—a person who was breathless, and panting on the least exertion —and had a certain share of those Nervous and Bilious Complaints, which are occasionally the companions of all who reside in great Cities—becomes enabled to run with ease and fleetness.

The Restorative Process having proceeded with healthful regularity—every part of the Constitution is effectively invigorated—a Man feels so conscious of the actual augmentation of all his powers, both Bodily and Mental, that he will undertake with alacrity—a task which before he shrunk from encountering.

The clearness of THE COMPLEXION is considered the *best criterion of a Man's being in good condition*—to which we add the appearance of the UNDER-LIP —which is plump and rosy, in proportion to the healthy plethora of the constitution:—this is a much more certain symptom of vigorous Health than any indication you can form from the appearance of the Tongue—or the PULSE, which is another very uncertain and deceiving Index,—the strength and frequency of which, not only varies in different persons, but in the same person in different circumstances and positions;—in some Irritable Constitutions *the vibration of the Heart varies almost as often as it Beats*— when we walk—stand—sit—or lie down—early in the morning—late in the evening—elated with good news—depressed by bad, &c.—when the Stomach is empty—after taking food—after a full meal of Nutritive food— after a spare one of *Maigre materials*. Moreover, it is impossible to ascertain the degree of deviation from Health by feeling a Pulse—unless we are well acquainted with the peculiarity of it, when the patient is in Health.

The Editor has now arrived at the most difficult part of his work, and needs all the assistance that Training can give, to excite him to proceed with any hope of developing the subject, with that perspicuity and effect—which it deserves, and he desires to give it.

The *Food—Clothes—Fire—Air—Exercise—Sleep—Wine*, &c. which may be most advisable for invigorating the Health of one individual—may be by no means the best adapted to produce a like good effect with another;—at the time of Life most people arrive at, before they think about these things —they are often become the slaves of habits which have grown with their growth, and strengthened with their strength—and the utmost that can be done after our 40th year, is to endeavour very gradually to correct them.

We caution those who are past the Meridian of Life (see *Index*)—to beware of suddenly abandoning established Customs, (especially of diminishing the warmth of their Clothing, or the nutritive quality of what they Eat and Drink), which, by long usage, often become as indispensable, as a Mathematical Valetudinarian reckoned his Flannel Waistcoat was—"in the *ratio* that my *Body* would be uncomfortable without my *Skin*—would my *Skin* be, without my *Flannel Waistcoat.*"

We recommend those who are in search of Health and Strength, to read the remarks which are classed under the titles WINE,—SIESTA,—CLOTHES, —"AIR"—"FIRE"—SLEEP—PEPTIC PRECEPTS, &c.

With the greatest deference, we submit the following sketch, to be variously modified by the Medical Adviser—according to the season of the Year—the Age—Constitution—and previous habits of the Patient,—the purpose it is intended to accomplish—or the Disorder it is intended to prevent or cure.

The first thing to be done, is to put the Principal Viscera into a condition to absorb the *pabulum vitæ*, we put into the Stomach—as much depends on the state of the Organs of Digestion[9] as on the quality of our Diet:— therefore commence with taking, early in the morning, fasting, about half an hour before Breakfast, about two drams of *Epsom Salts* (*i. e.* as much as will move the Bowels twice, not more,) in half a pint of warm water.—See *Index*.

The following day, go into a *Tepid Bath*, heated to about 95 degrees of *Fahrenheit*.

The Third day, take another dose of Salts—keeping to a light diet of Fish— Broths, &c. (Nos. 490, 563, 564, and 572). During the next week, take the TONIC TINCTURE, as directed in (No. 569). See *Index*. Thus far—any person may proceed without any difficulty,—and great benefit will he derive therefrom, if he cannot pursue the following part of the System:—

RISE early—if the Weather permits, amuse yourself with Exercise in the open air for some time before BREAKFAST—the material for which, I leave entirely to the previous habit of the Individual.

Such is the sensibility of the Stomach, when recruited by a good night's rest, that of all alterations in Diet, it will be most disappointed at any change of this Meal—either of the time it is taken—or of the quantity, or quality of it—so much so, that the functions of a delicate Stomach will be frequently deranged throughout the whole Day after.

The BREAKFAST I recommend, is Good Milk Gruel (No. 572), see *Index*, or Beef Tea (No. 563), see *Index*, or Portable Beef Tea (No. 252); a pint of the latter may be made for two-pence halfpenny, as easily as a Basin of Gruel.

The interval between *Breakfast* and *Eleven* o'clock, is the best time for Intellectual business—then *Exercise* again till about *Twelve*—when probably the Appetite will be craving for a LUNCHEON, which may consist of a bit of roasted Poultry,—a basin of good Beef Tea, or Eggs poached, (No. 546), or boiled in the Shell, (No. 547), Fish plainly dressed, (No. 144, or 145, &c.), or a Sandwich (No. 504),—stale Bread—and half a pint of good Home-brewed Beer—or Toast and Water, (No. 463*),—see *Index*,—with about one-fourth or one-third part of its measure of Wine, of which Port is preferred.

The solidity of the LUNCHEON should be proportionate to the time it is intended to enable you to wait for your Dinner, and the activity of the Exercise you take in the mean-time.

Take Exercise and Amusement as much as is convenient in the open air again, till past Four—then rest, and prepare for DINNER at *Five*—which should be confined to One Dish, of roasted Beef (No. 19), or Mutton (No. 23), five days in the week—boiled meat one—and roasted Poultry one—with a portion of sufficiently boiled ripe Vegetables—mashed Potatoes are preferred, see (No. 106), and the other fourteen ways of dressing this useful root.

The same restrictions from other articles of Food[10], as we have already mentioned in the plan for Training—*i. e.* if the person trained—has not arrived at that time of Life, when habit has become so strong—that to deprive him of those accustomed Indulgencies, &c. by which his health has hitherto been supported—would be as barbarous—as to take away Crutches from the Lame.

DRINK at Dinner, a pint of home-brewed Beer, or Toast and Water (No. 463*), with one-third or one-fourth part Wine, and a few glasses of Wine after—the less, the better—but take as much as custom has made necessary to excite that degree of circulation in your system, without which, you are uncomfortable. Read *Obs. on* "WINE."

AFTER DINNER sit quiet for a couple of hours—the *Semi-Siesta* is a pleasant position—*i. e.* the Feet on a stool about eight inches high,—or if your Exercise has fatigued you, lie down, and indulge in Horizontal Refreshment[11]:—this you may sometimes do with advantage before Dinner, if you have taken more Exercise than usual, and you feel tired:—when the Body is fatigued, the Stomach, by sympathy, will, in proportion, be incapable of doing its business of Digestion.

AT SEVEN, a little Tea, or warmed Milk with a very little Rum, a bit of Sugar, and a little Nutmeg in it—after which, Exercise and Amusement again, if convenient, in the open air.

For SUPPER, a Biscuit, or a Sandwich, (No. 504), or a bit of cold Fowl, &c. and a glass of Beer, or Wine, and Toast and Water (No. 463*),—and occasionally (No. 572), *i. e. as light a Supper as possible*—the sooner after *Ten* you retire to rest, the better.

For those who Dine very late—the best Supper is Gruel (No. 572), or a little Bread and Cheese, or Pounded Cheese (No. 542), and a glass of Beer —but if You have had an early, or a *Ban Yan Dinner*—or Instinct suggests that the exhaustion, from extraordinary exertion, requires more restorative materials,—furnish your Stomach with a Chop or a Chicken, &c. or some of the easily digestible and nutritive materials referred to in the *Index* under the article *Food for Feeble Stomachs*—and as much diffusible stimulus as will animate the Circulation, and ensure the influence of "Nature's sweet restorer, Balmy Sleep,"—the soundness of which,—depends entirely on the Stomach being in good temper, and the Heart supporting the circulation with Salutary Vigour. See the *Art of Sleeping.—Index.*

For the Diet to be confined to Beef and Mutton, is a sufficient abridgment of the amusements of the Mouth—it is a barbarous mortification, to insist on these being always cooked the same way[12], and we advise an occasional indulgence in the whole range of plain Cookery, from (No. 1) to (No. 98).

Broils (No. 94) are ordered in the plan for Training, probably, because the most convenient manner of obtaining the desired portion *Hot*,—(Food is then most easy of Digestion—*before the process of Digestion can commence, it must take the temperature of the Stomach*—which, when in a languid state, has no superfluous Heat to spare—) but as the Lean part is often scorched and dried, and the Fat becomes empyreumatic, from being in immediate contact with the Fire—a slice of well roasted Ribs (No. 20),—or Sir Loin of Beef (No. 19), or a Leg, Neck, Loin, or Saddle of Mutton (No. 23, or 26, or 31), must be infinitely more succulent and nutritive—whether this be rather *over*, or *under*-done, the previous habits of the Eater must determine—the Medium, between *over* and *under*-dressing—is in general most Agreeable, and certainly most Wholesome.

That *Meat* which is considerably *under*-done, contains more Nutriment than that which is *over*-done, is true enough;—that which is *not done at all*, contains a great deal more—but, in the ratio that it is *Raw*[13], so is it unfortunately difficult of digestion, as *Spallanzani* (see *Index*) has proved by actual and satisfactory experiments.

OUR FOOD MUST BE DONE—*either by our Cook,—or by our Stomach,—*before Digestion can take place—(see 1st page of *Obs.* on *Siesta*); surely no man in his senses, would willingly be so wanting in consideration of the comfort, &c. of his Stomach, as to give it the needless trouble of Cooking and Digesting also—and waste its valuable energies in work which a Spit or a Stewpan can do better.

Thoroughly dressed BEEF (No. 19), or MUTTON (No. 23), is incomparably the most animating Food we can furnish our Stomachs with, and sound HOME-BREWED BEER, the most invigorating Drink—It is indeed, Gentle Reader, notwithstanding a foolish fashion has banished the natural beverage of Great Britain—as extremely ungenteel.—

> "Your Wine tippling, Dram sipping fellows retreat,
> But your Beer-drinking Briton can never be beat."

The best Tests of the Restorative qualities of Food—are a small quantity of it satisfying Hunger,—the strength of the Pulse after it,—and the length of Time which elapses before Appetite returns again:—according to these Rules, the Editor's own experience gives a decided verdict in favour of

Roasted or Broiled Beef (No. 19 or 94), or Mutton (No. 26 or 23), as most nutritive,—then Game and Poultry, of which the meat is Brown, (No. 59, or 61, or 74), next Veal and Lamb and Poultry, of which the meat is White—the Fat kinds of Fish, Eels—Salmon—Herrings, &c. and least nutritive, the white kinds of Fish—such as Whiting, Cod, Soles, Haddocks, &c. For further information, see *Oysters*, (No. 181).

The celebrated Trainer, Sir Thomas Parkyns, &c., "greatly preferred BEEF-EATERS—to *Sheep-biters*, as they called those who ate Mutton."

By DR. STARK'S *very curious Experiments on Diet*, p. 110, it appears, that "when he fed upon *Roasted Goose*, he was much more vigorous both in Body and Mind, than with any other food."

That *Fish* is less nutritive than FLESH—the speedy return of Hunger after a dinner of Fish is sufficient proof—when a Trainer at Newmarket[14] wishes *to waste a Jockey*—he is not allowed *Pudding*, if Fish can be had.

Crabs,—Lobsters (No. 176), Prawns, &c. unless thoroughly boiled, (which those sold ready boiled seldom are), are tremendously indigestible.

Shell Fish have long held a high rank in the catalogue of easily digestible and speedily restorative Foods:—of these *Oysters* (No. 181), certainly deserve the best character; but we think that they, as well as *Eggs,—Gelatinous Substances,—Rich Broths*[15], &c. have acquired not a little more reputation for these qualities than they deserve.

OYSTERS are often cold and uncomfortable to Dyspeptic Stomachs—unless warmed with a certain quantity of Pepper, and good White Wine.

To recruit the Animal Spirits, and produce Strength, there is nothing like BEEF and MUTTON—moreover, when kept till properly tender, none will give less trouble to the Digestive organs—and more substantial excitement to the Constitution.

The Editor has dined for some years principally upon plainly roasted or boiled Beef and Mutton, and has often observed, that if he changes it for any other Food for several days together—that he suffers a diminution of strength, &c. and is disposed on such days to drink an additional Glass of *Wine*, &c. See *Index*.

However, the fitness of various Foods, and Drinks—and the quantity of Nutriment which they afford—depends very much upon how they are prepared, and as much on the inclination and abilities of the concoctive faculties, which have the task of converting them into Chyle.

It is quite as absurd, to suppose, that one kind of Diet, &c. is equally adapted to every kind of Constitution—as that one Remedy will cure all Diseases.

To produce the highest degree of Health and Strength—we must supply the Stomach with not merely that material which contains the greatest quantity of Nourishment—but in making our reckoning, must take into the account, the degree in which it is adapted to the habits and powers of the Organ which is to digest it—the Arms of a Giant are of little use in the Hands of a Dwarf.

The Plan we have proposed, was calculated for Midsummer-day,—when plenty of hard Exercise in the open Air will soon create an Appetite for the substantial Diet we have recommended—it is taken for granted, that a Person has the opportunity of devoting a couple of months to the re-establishment of his Health—and that during that time, he will be content to consider himself in the same state as any other Animal out of condition—and disposed to submit cheerfully to such a modification of the rules recommended, as his Medical Adviser may deem most convenient to the circumstances of the Case, and the Age, the Constitution, and previous habits of the Patient, &c. &c.

Every part of this system must be observed in proportion—and EXERCISE increased in the same degree, that NOURISHMENT is introduced to the Constitution.

The best General Rule for Diet that I can write, is to Eat and Drink only of such Foods—at such times,—and in such quantities—as Experience has convinced you, agree with your Constitution—and absolutely to avoid all other.

A very different Regimen must be observed by those who live a Life with Labour—or Exercise—or of Indolence,—and at the different Periods of Life.

HUMAN LIFE may be divided into *Three Stages*.

The FIRST, *The period of Preparation* from our birth, till about our 21st year, when the Body has generally attained the *acmé* of expansion:—till then, a continual and copious supply of Chyle is necessary, not only to keep our machinery in repair, but to furnish material for the increase of it.

The SECOND from 21 to 42, *The period of Active Usefulness*; during which, nothing more is wanted, than to restore the daily waste, occasioned by the actions of the Vital and Animal Functions.

The THIRD, *The period of Decline*: this comes on and proceeds with more or less celerity, according to the original strength of the Constitution, and the Economy[16] with which it has been managed during the second period. (Age is a relative term,—one man is as old at 40 as another is at 60): but after 42, the most vigorous become gradually more passive[17]—and after 63, pretty nearly quite so.

SIR WILLIAM JONES'S ANDROMETER.

	3	6	9	12	
1					—Ideas received through the Senses.
					—Speaking, and Pronunciation.
					—Letters, and Spelling.
					—Ideas retained in the Memory.
5					—Reading and Repeating.
					—Grammar of his own Language.
					—Memory exercised.
					—Moral and Religions Lessons.
					—Natural History and Experiments.
10					—Dancing, Music, Drawing, Exercises.
					—History of his own Country.
					—Latin.
					—Greek.
					—French and Italian.
15					—Translations.
					—Compositions in Verse and Prose.
					—Rhetoric and Declamation.
					—History and Law.
					—Logic and Mathematics.
20					—Rhetorical Exercises.
					—Philosophy and Politics.
					—Compositions in his own Language.
					—Declamations continued.
					—Ancient Orators studied.

25		—Travel and Conversation.
		—Speeches at the Bar, or in Parliament.
		—State Affairs.
		—Historical Studies continued.
		—Law and Eloquence.
30		—Public Life.
		—Private and Social Virtues.
		—Habits of Eloquence improved.
		—Philosophy resumed at leisure.
		—Orations published.
35		—Exertions in State and Parliament.
		—Civil Knowledge mature.
		—Eloquence perfect.
		—National Rights defended.
		—The Learned protected.
40		—The Virtuous assisted.
		—Compositions published.
		—Science improved.
		—Parliamentary Affairs.
		—Laws enacted, and supported.
45		—Fine Arts patronized.
		—Government of his Family.
		—Education of his Children.
		—Vigilance as a Magistrate.
		—Firmness as a Patriot.
50		—Virtue as a Citizen.
		—Historical Works.
		—Oratorical Works.
		—Philosophical Works.
		—Political Works.
55		—Mathematical Works.
		}
		}
		}Continuation of former Pursuits.
		}
60		}
		—Fruits of his Labour enjoyed.
		—A glorious Retirement.
		—An amiable Family.
		—Universal Respect.
65		—Consciousness of a Virtuous Life.
		}
		}
		}*Perfection of Earthly Happiness.*
		}

The most common cause of Dyspeptic Disorders, which are so prevalent at the commencement of the Third Period of Life—is an increasing indolence, inducing us to diminish the degree of the active Exercise we have been in the habit of taking—without in a corresponding degree diminishing the quantity of our Food—on the contrary, people seem to expect the Stomach to grow stronger and to work harder as it gets Older, and to almost entirely support the Circulation without the help of Exercise.—

As the activity of our existence—and the accommodating powers of the Stomach, &c. diminish—in like degree—must we lessen the quantity—and be careful of the quality of our Food, eat oftener and less at a time—or Indigestion—and the multitude of Disorders of which it is the fruitful parent, will soon destroy us.

The System of Cornaro has been oftener quoted, than understood—most people imagine, it was one of rigid Abstinence and comfortless Self-denial —but this was not the case:—his Code of Longevity consisted in steadily obeying the suggestions of Instinct—and Economizing his Vitality, and living under his income of Health,—carefully regulating his temper—and cultivating cheerful habits.

The following is a Compendium of his plan—*in his own words.*

He tells us that *when Fourscore*

"I am used to take in all twelve ounces of solid nourishment, such as Meat, and the yolk of an Egg, &c. and fourteen ounces of drink:—I eat Bread, Soup, New-laid Eggs, Veal, Kid, Mutton, Partridge, Pullets, Pigeons, &c. and some Sea and River Fish.

"I made choice of such Wines and Meats as agreed with my Constitution, and declined all other diet—and proportioned the quantity thereof to the strength of my Stomach, and abridged my Food—as my years increased.

"Every one is the best judge of the food which is most agreeable to his own Stomach,—it is next to impossible, to judge what is best for another;—the Constitutions of men are as different from each other as their complexions."—p. 36.

"1st. Take care of the quality.

"2dly. Of the quantity—so as to eat and drink nothing that offends the Stomach, nor any more than you can easily digest: your experience ought to be your guide in these two principles when you arrive at *Forty*: by that time you ought to know that you are in the midst of your life; thanks to the goodness of your Constitution which has carried you so far: but that when you are arrived to this period, you go down the hill apace—and it is necessary for you to change your course of life, especially with regard to the quantity and quality of your diet—because it is on that, the health and length of our days do radically depend. Lastly; if the former part of our lives has been altogether sensual—the latter ought to be rational and regular; order being necessary for the preservation of all things, especially the life of man.—Longevity cannot be attained without continence and sobriety[18]."

> "At *thirty* Man suspects himself a Fool,
> Knows it at *forty,* and reforms his plan."

By the small quantity of Food, and great proportion of his Meat to his Drink, this noble Venetian, at the age of *forty,* freed himself, by the advice of his Physicians, from several grievous disorders contracted by intemperance, and lived in health of body, and great cheerfulness of mind, to above an hundred.—Briefly, the secret of his Longevity seems to have been, a gradually increasing Temperance "in omnibus"—and probably, after a certain time of Life, abstinence from the "opus magnum."

The source of physical and moral Health, Happiness, and Longevity,—

> "Reason's whole pleasure, all the Joys of Sense
> Lie in three words, Health, peace, and competence.
> But Health consists in temperance alone;
> And Peace, oh Virtue! Peace is all thy own."
>   POPE.

Intensive Life, can only be purchased at the price of *Extensive.*

If you force the Heart to gallop as fast during the second, as it does during the first stage of life—and make the steady fire of 42, to blaze as brightly as the flame of 21,—it will very soon be burnt out.

Those who cannot be content to submit to that diminution of action ordained by nature, against which there is no appeal,—as it is the absolute covenant, by the most attentive and implicit observance of which we can only hope to hold our lease of life comfortably,—will soon bring to the diminished energy of the Second Stage of Life—the Paralysis of the Third.

From 40 to 60, a witty French author tells us, is *"La belle saison[19] pour la Gourmandise;"*—for the artificial pleasures of the Palate, it may be, and the *Bon Vivant* cultivates them as the means of prolonging the vigour of Youth —and procrastinating the approach of Age.

Restoration may certainly be considerably facilitated, by preparing and dressing food so as to render it easily soluble—if the secret of Rejuvenization be ever discovered; it will be found in the Kitchen.

Very soon after we pass the *Meridian of Life*, (which, according to those who train men for athletic exercises, and to Dr. Jameson,[20] is our 28th, and to Dr. Cheyne, about our 35th year,) the elasticity of the Animal System imperceptibly diminishes,—our Senses become less susceptible, and are every hour getting the worse for wear, however Self-Love, assisted by your Hair-dresser, and Tailor, &c. may endeavour to persuade you to the contrary.

Digestion and Sleep are less perfect—the restorative process more and more fails to keep pace with the consuming process—the body is insufficiently repaired, more easily deranged, and with more difficulty brought into adjustment again; till at length the vital power being diminished, and the organs deteriorated,—Nourishment can neither be received, or prepared and diffused through the constitution—and Consumption so much exceeds Renovation, that decay rapidly closes the scene of Life.

One may form some Idea of *the Self-consumption of the human body*, by reflecting that the pulsation of the Heart, and the motion of the Blood connected with it, takes place 100,000 times every day; *i. e.* on an average

the pulse[21] beats	70	times in a minute,
multiplied by	60	minutes in an hour,
	————	
	4200	
	24	hours in a day,
	————	
	16800	
	8400	
	————	
	100800	pulsations in a day.

What Machine, of the most adamantine material, will not soon be the worse for wear, from such incessant vibration—especially if the Mainsprings of it are not preserved in a state of due regulation?

The generative faculties, which are the last that Nature finishes—are the first that fail.—Economy in the exercise of them—especially before and after the second period of Life—is the grand precept for the restoration and accumulation of Strength, the preservation of Health, and the prolongation of Life;—we are vigorous, in proportion to the perfection of the performance of the Restorative process, *i. e.* as we Eat hearty, and Sleep soundly—as our Body loses the power of renovating itself, in like ratio, fails its faculty of creating—what may be a salutary subduction of the superfluous health of the Second—during the Third period of life, will be a destructive sacrifice of the strength of both the Mind and the Body.—See also the 9th chapter of the *First* Edition of WILLICH *on Diet.* 8vo. 1799.

The next organical defect, (we perceive too plainly for our self-love to mistake it,) is manifested by THE EYE[22]. To read a small print—you must remove it from the Eye further than you have been accustomed to do—and place it in a better light.

The FALSETTO Voice now begins to fail, and THE EAR loses some of its quickness—several extraordinary Musicians have been able till then, if a handful of the keys of a Harpsichord were put down so as to produce the most irrelative combinations—to name each half note without a mistake.— When I mentioned this to that excellent Organ Player, Mr. Charles Wesley, he said, "At the age of twenty, I could do it myself—but I can't now." He was then in his 55th year.

About the same time, the Palate is no longer contented with being employed as a mere shovel to the Stomach,—and as it finds its master becomes every day more difficult to please—learns to be a more watchful Purveyor.

After 40,—the strongest People begin to talk about being *Bilious,* or *Nervous,* &c. &c. and the Stomach will no longer do its duty properly— unless the Food offered to it is perfectly agreeable to it—when offended, *Indigestion* brings with it, all that melancholy depression of the Animal Spirits, which disables a Man from either thinking with precision, or acting with vigour—during the distressing suspension of the restorative process— arise all those miseries of Mind and Body, which drive Fools to get drunk, and make Madmen commit suicide:—without due attention to Diet, &c. the Third period of Life is little better than a Chronic Disease.

As our assimilating powers become enfeebled, we must endeavour to entertain them with food so prepared, as to give them the least trouble, and the most nourishment[23].

In the proportion that our Food is restorative, and properly digested—our bodies are preserved in Health and Strength—and all our faculties continue vigorous and perfect.

If it is unwholesome, ill-prepared, and indigestible—the Body languishes, and is exhausted even in its youth—its strength and faculties daily decrease, and it sinks beneath the weight of the painful sensations attendant on a state of Decay.

Would to Heaven that a Cook could help our Stomachs, as much as an Optician can our Eyes: our Existence would be as much more perfect than it now is, as our Sight is superior to our other Senses.

"The vigour of the Mind decays with that of the Body—and not only Humour and Invention, but even Judgment and Resolution, change and languish, with ill constitution of Body and of Health."—Sir WILLIAM TEMPLE.

The following account of the successful REDUCTION OF CORPULENCE AND IMPROVEMENT OF HEALTH, the Editor can vouch for being a faithful statement of Facts.

30 January, 1821.

MY DEAR SIR,

In consequence of the Conversation I had with you, upon the advantages I had derived from Exercise and attention to Diet in the reduction of Weight, and your desire that I should communicate as far as I recollect them, the particulars of my Case; I have great pleasure in forwarding to you the following Statement.

I measure in height six Feet and half an Inch,—possess a sound Constitution and considerable activity.—At *the age of Thirty* I weighed about 18 Stone—two years afterwards I had reached the great weight of nineteen Stone, in perfect Health, always sleeping well and enjoying good Appetite and Spirits—soon after, however, I began to experience the usual attendants on fullness of Habit, a disinclination to rise in the morning from drowsiness, heaviness about the Forehead after I had risen, and a disposition to Giddiness;—I was also attacked by a complaint in one of my Eyes, the Symptoms of which it is unnecessary to describe, but it proved to be occasioned by fullness of blood, as it was removed by cupping in the temple. I lost four ounces of blood from the temple; and thinking that the loss of a little more might be advantageous, I had eight ounces taken from the back; and in order to prevent the necessity, as far as possible, of future bleeding, I resolved to reduce the system—by increasing my Exercise and diminishing my Diet.

I therefore took an early opportunity of seeing Mr. Jackson, (whose respectability and skill as a teacher of sparring is universally acknowledged,) and after some Conversation with him, determined upon acting under his Advice.

I accordingly commenced *Sparring*, having provided myself with flannel Dresses, which I always used, being extremely careful on changing them to avoid the risk of cold, and I recollect no instance in which I was not successful.

I also had recourse to *Riding* Schools, riding without stirrups, so as to have the advantage of the most powerful exercise the Horse could give;—these exercises I took in the morning in the proportion probably of sparring twice a week, and riding three or four times.

Frequently at night I resumed my Exercise,—*Walking* and sometimes *Running*, generally performing about five miles an hour, till I again produced perspiration; every other Opportunity I could resort to of bodily exercise I also availed myself of.

In respect to diet, I had accustomed myself to Suppers and drinking excellent Table Beer in large quantities, and for probably ten Years, had indulged myself with Brandy and Water after Supper:—this practice I entirely discontinued, substituting Toast and Water with my Dinner, and Tea and a good allowance of Toast for Supper, always avoiding copious Draughts.

I left off drinking malt Liquor as a habit, and indeed, very seldom drank it at all.—I took somewhat less meat at Dinner, avoiding Pies and Puddings as much as possible, but always took three or four Glasses of Port after dinner.

During the time I was under this training, I took the opinion of an eminent Physician upon the subject, who entirely approved of my Plan, and recommended the occasional use of Aperient medicine, but which I seldom resorted to.

The Result of all this, was a reduction of my Weight of upwards of three Stone, or about Forty-five Pounds, *in about six or seven months.*—I found my activity very much increased, and my wind excellent, but, I think, my Strength not quite so great, though I did not experience any material Reduction of it: my Health was perfect throughout.

I then relaxed my System a little, and have up to the present time, being a period of ten Years, avoided the necessity of bleeding, and have enjoyed an almost uninterrupted continuance of good Health, although my Weight has gradually increased; sometimes, however, fluctuating between 7 or 8 Pounds and a Stone, according to my means of Exercise,—always increasing in Winter, and losing in Summer;—and at this moment (January 29th, 1821,) I am about a Stone more than I ought to be, having ascertained, that my best bodily Strength, is at sixteen Stone and a half.

When the object is *to Reduce Weight*, rest and moderate Food will always sufficiently restore the exhaustion arising from Exercise;—if an additional quantity of Food and nourishing Liquors be resorted to, the Body will in general be restored to the weight it was before the Exercise.

I have sometimes lost from ten ounces to a Pound in weight by an Hour's sparring. If the object be not to reduce the weight, the Food may safely be proportioned to the Exercise.

You will readily perceive, that the plan I adopted, ought only to be resorted to by Persons of sound Constitution and of athletic bodily Frame,—it would be absurd to lay down a general rule for the adoption of all fat men.

I think, with all lusty men, the drinking of malt Liquor of any kind is injurious,—Meat taken more than once a day is liable to the same Objection. I still persevere in the disuse of malt Liquors and Spirits, and Suppers, seldom taking more than four Glasses of Wine as a habit,—although I do not now deem it necessary to make myself so far the Slave of habit, as to refuse the Pleasures of the Table when they offer.

I am, dear Sir,

Yours very truly,

The following are the most interesting Facts in Dr. Bryan Robinson's Essay on the Food and Discharges of the Human Body, 8vo. 1748, which has become scarce.

"I am now, in *May* 1747, in the 68th year of my age. The length of my Body is 63 Inches: I am of a sanguine but not robust constitution—and am at present neither lean nor fat. In the year 1721 the Morning weight of my body without Clothes, was about 131 Avoirdupois pounds, the daily weight of my food at a medium was about 85 Avoirdupois ounces, and the proportion of my Drink to my Meat, I judge was at that time about 2.5—to 1.

"At the latter end of *May* 1744, my weight was above 164 pounds, and the proportion of my Drink to my Meat was considerably greater than before, and had been so for some time. I was then seized with a Paralytic disorder, which obliged me to make an alteration in my diet. In order to settle the proportion of my Drink to my Meat, I considered what others have said concerning this proportion.

"According to *Sanctorius*, though he reckons it a disproportion, the drink to the meat in his time, was about 10 to 3 in temperate bodies.

CORNARO's drink to his Meat, was as	7 to 6.
Mr. RYE's, in winter, as	4 to 3.
Dr. LINING's, at a medium	11 to 3.
And my drink to my meat	5 to 2.
A mean taken from all these makes the Drink to the Meat—about	2 to 1.

B. ROBINSON *on Food and Discharges*, p. 34.

"At the age of 64, by lessening my food, and increasing the proportion of my meat to my drink, *i. e.* by lessening my drink about a third part, (*i. e.* to 20 ounces) and my meat about a sixth, (*i. e.* 38 ounces) of what they were in 1721, I have freed myself for these two years past from the returns of a *Sore throat* and *Diarrhœa,*—Disorders I often had, though they were but slight, and never confined me. I have been much more costive than I was before, when I lived more fully, and took more Exercise, and have greatly, for my age, recovered the paralytic weakness I was seized with three years ago.

"Hence we gather, that good and constant Health consists in a just quantity of food; and a just proportion of the meat to the drink: and that to be freed from chronical disorders contracted by Intemperance—the quantity of food ought to be lessened; and the proportion of the meat to the drink increased —more or less, according to the greatness of the disorders, p. 61.

"I commonly ate four ounces of Bread and Butter, and drank half a pound of a very weak infusion of Green Tea for *Breakfast*. For *Dinner* I took two ounces of Bread, and the rest Flesh-meat,—Beef, Mutton, Pork, Veal, Hare, Rabbit, Goose, Turkey, Fowl tame and wild, and Fish. I generally chose the strongest meats as fittest, since they agreed well with my stomach, to keep up the power of my body under this great diminution of my food; I seldom took any *Garden stuff*—finding that it commonly lessened perspiration and *increased my weight*.—I drank four ounces of water with my meat and a pound of Claret after I had done eating. At night I ate nothing, but drank 12 ounces of water with a pipe of Tobacco, p. 63.

"There is but one Weight, under which a grown body can enjoy the best and most uninterrupted Health. p. 91. That Weight is such as enables the Heart to supply the several parts of the body with just quantities of Blood. p. 100.

"The weight under which an Animal has the greatest strength and activity— which I shall call its *Athletic weight*,—is that weight under which the Heart —and the proportion of the weight of the Heart to the weight of the body are greatest: the strength of the Muscles is measured by the strength of the Heart, p. 117.

"If the weight of the body of an Animal be greater than its *Athletic Weight*, it may be reduced to that weight by evacuations, dry food and exercise. These lessen the weight of the Body, by wasting its fat, and lessening its Liver; and they increase the weight of the Heart, by increasing the quantity and motion of the blood. Thus a game Cock in ten days is reduced to his athletic weight, and prepared for fighting.

"If the Food, which with Evacuations and Exercise, reduced the Cock to his athletic weight in ten days, be continued any longer, the Cock will not have that strength and activity which he had before under his athletic weight;

which may be owing to the loss of weight going on after he arrives at his athletic weight.

"It is known by experiment, that a Cock cannot stand above 24 hours at his athletic weight, and that a Cock has changed very much for the worse in 12 hours.

"When a Cock is at the top of his condition, that is, when he is at his athletic weight, his Head is of a glowing red colour, his Neck thick, and his Thigh thick and firm;—the day after his complexion is less glowing, his Neck thinner, and his Thigh softer;—and the third day his Thigh will be very soft and flaccid. p. 119.

"If the increase of weight in a small compass of time, rise to above a certain quantity, it will cause disorders.

"I can bear an increase of above a pound and a half in one day, and an increase of three or four pounds in six or seven days, without being disordered; but think I should suffer from an increase of five or six pounds in that time.

"An increase of weight may be carried off by lessening the Food,—or by increasing the Discharges.—The discharges may be increased either by exercise, or by evacuations procured by art.

"By lessening the daily quantity of my food to 23 ounces, I have lost 26 ounces;—by fasting a whole day, I lost 48 ounces, having gained 27 the day before.

"Mr. Rye was a strong, well set, corpulent man, of a sanguine complexion; by a brisk walk for one hour before breakfast he threw off, by insensible perspiration, one pound of increased weight; by a walk of three hours, he threw off two pounds of increased weight. The best way to take off an increase of weight which threatens a distemper, is either by fasting or exercise. p. 84.

"The mean loss of weight by several grown bodies caused by a purging medicine composed of a drachm of *Jalap* and ten grains of *Calomel*, was about 2¾ Avoirdupois pounds; and the mean quantity of Liquor, drank during the time of Purging, was about double the loss of Weight."— ROBINSON *on the Animal Economy*, p. 458.

"I have lost, by a spontaneous *Diarrhœa*, two pounds in twenty-four hours; and Mr. Rye lost twice that quantity in the same time."—*On the Food and Discharges of Human Bodies*, by B. ROBINSON, p. 84.

"Most *Chronic Diseases*—arise from too much *Food* and too little *Exercise*, —both of which lessen the weight of the Heart and the quantity of Blood;— the first by causing fatness; the second by a diminution of the blood's motion.

"Hence, when the LIVER is grown too large by Intemperance and Inactivity, it may be lessened and brought to a healthful magnitude by Temperance and Exercise.—It may be emptied other ways by art; but nothing can prevent its filling again, and consequently secure good and constant Health—but an exact Diet and Exercise. Purging and Vomiting may lessen the Liver, and reduce it to its just magnitude;—but these evacuations cannot prevent its increasing again, so long as persons live too fully, and use too little exercise —and can only be done by lessening the Food and increasing the Exercise.

"Much sleep, much food, and little exercise, are the principal things which make animals grow fat. If the Body, on account of Age or other Infirmities, cannot use sufficient Exercise, and takes much the same quantity of Sleep, its weight must be lessened by lessening the Food, which may be done by lessening the Drink, without making any change in the Meat; as I have proved myself by experience."—p. 90.

On this subject, see also—Dr. STARK on *Diet*, and SANCTORIUS' *Medecina Statica*. Dr. HEMING on *Corpulency*.—Mr. WADD on *Corpulency*.—Dr. ARBUTHNOT on *Aliment*.

SLEEP.

"When tired with vain rotations of the Day,
Sleep winds us up for the succeeding dawn."

YOUNG.

Health may be as much injured by interrupted and *insufficient Sleep,* as by luxurious indulgence.

Valetudinarians who regularly retire to rest, and arise at certain hours, are unable, without injurious violence to their feelings—to resist the inclination to do so.

"Pliant Nature more or less demands
As Custom forms her; and *all sudden change*
She hates, of Habit even from *bad* to *good.*
If faults in Life—or new emergencies
From Habits[24] urge you by *long time* confirm'd,
Slow must the change arrive, and stage by stage,
Slow as the stealing progress of the Year."

ARMSTRONG'S *Art of Preserving Health.*

How important it is, then, to cultivate good and convenient Habits:— *Custom* will soon render the most rigid rules, not only easy, but agreeable.

—

"The Strong, by bad habits, grow weaker, we know;
And by good ones, the Weak will grow stronger also."

The Debilitated require much more rest than the Robust:—nothing is so restorative to the nerves, as sound, and uninterrupted Sleep, which is the chief source of both Bodily and Mental Strength.

The Studious need a full portion of Sleep, which seems to be as necessary nutriment to the Brain, as Food is to the Stomach.

Our Strength and Spirits are infinitely more exhausted by the exercise of our Mental, than by the labour of our Corporeal faculties—let any person try the effect of *Intense Application* for a few hours—He will soon find how much his Body is fatigued thereby, although He has not stirred from the Chair He sat on.

Those who are candidates for Health—must be as circumspect in the task they set their mind,—as in the exercise they give to their Body.

Dr. ARMSTRONG, the Poet of Health, observes,

"'Tis *the great Art of* LIFE to manage well
The restless Mind."

The grand secret seems to be, to contrive that the exercise of the Body, and that of the Mind, may serve as relaxations to each other.

Over Exertion, or Anxiety of Mind, disturbs Digestion infinitely more than any fatigue of Body—the Brain demands a much more abundant supply of the Animal Spirits, than is required for the excitement of mere Legs and Arms.

"'Tis the Sword that wears out the Scabbard."

Of the two ways of fertilizing the Brain—by Sleep, or by Spirituous Stimulus—(for some write best in the Morning, others when wound up with Wine, after Dinner or Supper:) the former is much less expensive—and less injurious to the constitution than either Port, or Brandy, whose aid it is said that some of our best Authors have been indebted to, for their most brilliant productions.

Calling one day on a literary friend, we found him reclining on a Sofa—on expressing our concern to find him indisposed, he said, "No, I was only *hatching,*—I have been writing till I was quite tired—my paper must go to Press to day—so I was taking my usual restorative—*A Nap*—which if it only lasts five minutes, so refreshes my Mind—that my Pen goes to work again spontaneously."

Is it not better *Economy of Time*, to go to sleep for half an hour,—than to go on noodling all day in a nerveless and semi-superannuated state—if not asleep, certainly not effectively Awake—for any purpose requiring the Energy of either the Body, or the Mind.

"*A Forty Winks Nap*," in an horizontal posture, is the best preparative for any extraordinary exertion of either.

Those who possess, and employ the powers of the Mind most—seldom attain the greatest Age[25]:—see BRUNAUD *de L'Hygiene des Gens de Lettres, Paris*, 8vo. 1819:—the Envy their Talent excites,—the Disappointment they often meet with in their expectations of receiving the utmost attention and respect, (which the world has seldom the gratitude to pay them while they live,) keep them in a perpetual state of irritation and disquiet—which frets them prematurely to their Grave[26].

To rest a whole Day—under great fatigue of either Body or Mind, is occasionally extremely beneficial—it is impossible to regulate Sleep by the hour;—when the Mind and the Body have received all the refreshment which Sleep can give, people cannot lie in Bed, and till then, they should not Rise[27].

> "Preach not me your musty Rules
>   Ye Drones, that mould in idle cell;
> The Heart is wiser than the Schools,
>   The Senses always reason well."
>   COMUS.

Our Philosophical Poet here gives the best practical maxim on the subject for Valetudinarians—who, by following his advice, may render their Existence, instead of a dull unvaried round of joyless, useless self-denial,—a circle of agreeable sensation;—for instance, go not to your Bed till You are tired of sitting up—then remain in an Horizontal posture,—till You long to change it for a Vertical: thus, by a little management, the inevitable business of Life may be converted into a source of continual Enjoyment.

All-healing Sleep soon neutralizes the corroding caustic of Care—and blunts even the barbed arrows of the marble-hearted Fiend, Ingratitude.

When the Pulse is almost paralysed by Anxiety,—half an hour's repose, will cheer the circulation, restore tranquillity to the perturbed spirit—and dissipate those heavy clouds of *Ennui*, which sometimes threaten to eclipse the brightest Minds, and best Hearts.—Child of Woe, lay thy Head on thy pillow, (instead of thy Mouth to the bottle,) and bless me for directing Thee to the true source of Lethe—and most sovereign *Nepenthé* for the Sorrows of Human Life.

The Time requisite to restore the waste occasioned by the action of the Day —depends on the activity of the habits, and on the Health of the Individual, —in general it cannot be less than Seven—and need not be more than Nine hours[28].

Invalids will derive much benefit from indulging in the *Siesta* whenever they feel languid.

A Sailor will tell you, that a Seaman can sleep as much in five hours, as a Landsman can in ten.

Whether rising very early lengthens Life we know not,—but think that sitting up very late shortens it,—and recommend you to rise by eight, and retire to rest by eleven; your feelings will bear out the adage, that "*one* Hour's rest before midnight, is worth *two* after."

When OLD PEOPLE have been examined with a view to ascertain the causes of their Longevity, they have uniformly agreed in one thing only,—that they ALL *went to Bed early, and rose early*.

> "Early to bed, and early to rise,
> Will make you healthy, wealthy, and wise."

Dr. FRANKLIN published an ingenious Essay on the advantage of early rising —He called it "*an Economical Project*," and calculated, that the saving that might be made in the City of Paris, *by using Sunshine instead of Candles*— at no less than £4,000,000 Sterling.

If the Delicate, and the nervous, the very Young, or the very Old—sit up beyond their usual hour, they feel the want of artificial aid, to raise their spirits to what is no more than the ordinary pitch of those who are in the vigour of their Life—and must fly from the festive board—or purchase a few hours of hilarity at the heavy price of Head-Ach and Dyspepsia for many days after; and a terrible exasperation of any Chronic Complaint they are afflicted with.

When the Body and Mind are both craving repose—to force their action, by the spur of spirituous stimulus, is the most extravagant waste of the "Vis Vitæ," that Fashion ever invented to consume her foolish Votaries—for Fools they certainly are, who mortgage the comfort of a Week, for the conviviality of an Hour—with the certainty of their term of Life being speedily foreclosed by Gout, Palsy, &c.

Among the most distressing miseries of this "Elysium of Bricks and Mortar," may be reckoned how rarely we enjoy "the sweets of a Slumber unbroke."

Sound passes through the thin PARTY WALLS of modern Houses, (*which of the first rate, at the* FIRE PLACE, *are only four inches in thickness*;) with most unfortunate facility; this is really an evil of the first magnitude,—if You are so unlucky as to have for next door neighbours—fashionable folks who turn night into day, or such as delight in the sublime Economy of Cindersaving, or Cobweb catching,—it is in vain to seek repose, before the former has indulged in the Evening's recreation of raking out the Fire, and has played with the Poker till it has made all the red coals black; or, after *Molidusta*, the Tidy One, has awoke the Morn—with "the Broom, the bonny, bonny Broom."

A determined Dusthunter, or Cindersaver, murders its neighbour's sleep—with as little mercy, as Macbeth did Malcolm's—and bangs doors, and rattles Window shutters, till the "Earth trembles, and Air is aghast!"

All attempts to conciliate a Savage who is in this fancy—will be labour in vain—the arrangement of its fire[29] is equally the occupation of the morning, and the amusement of the evening; the preservation of a Cinder and the destruction of a Cobweb, are the main business of its existence:— the best advice we can give you, gentle Reader—is to send it this little Book —and beseech it to place the following pages opposite to its Optic nerves some morning—after you have diverted it from Sleep every half hour during the preceding Night[30].

Counsellor SCRIBBLEFAST, a Special Pleader, who lived on a ground-floor in the Temple—about the time that Sergeant PONDER who dwelt on the first floor, retired to rest, began to practise his Violoncello, *"And his loud voice in Thunder spoke."*—The Student above—by way of giving him a gentle hint, struck up *"Gently strike the warbling Lyre,"* and Will. Harmony's favourite Hornpipes of *"Dont Ye,"* and *"Pray be Quiet:"* however, the *dolce* and *pianissimo* of poor PONDER produced no diminution of the *prestissimo* and *fortissimo* of the indefatigable SCRIBBLEFAST.

PONDER, prayed "silence in the Court," and complained in most pathetic terms—but, alas! his "LOWLY SUIT AND PLAINTIVE DITTY" made not the least impression on him who was beneath him.—He at length procured a set of Skettles, and as soon as his musical neighbour had done fiddling, he began *con strepito*, and bowled away merrily till the morning dawned.—The enraged Musician did not wait long after daylight, to put in his plea against such proceedings, and received in reply, that such exercise had been ordered by a Physician, as the properest Paregoric, after being disturbed by the thorough Bass of the Big Fiddle below—this soon convinced the tormentor of Catgut, who dwelt on the Ground-Floor, that He could not annoy his superior with Impunity, and produced silence on both sides.

People are very unwisely inconsiderate how much it is their own Interest to attend to the comforts of their Neighbours, for which we have a divine command "to love our neighbour as ourself." *"Sic utere tuo, ut alienum non lædas,"* is the maxim of our English law. Interrupting one's Sleep is as prejudicial to Health, as any of the nuisances Blackstone enumerates as actionable.

The majority of the *Dogs,—Parrots,—Piano-Fortes*, &c. in this Metropolis, are *Actionable Nuisances*!!!

However inferior in rank and fortune, &c. your next door neighbour may be —there are moments when He may render you the most valuable service. —"A Lion owed his life to the exertions of a Mouse."

Those who have not the power to please—should have the discretion not to offend;—the most humble may have opportunities to return a Kindness, or resent an Insult.

It is Madness to wantonly annoy any one.

There is plenty of Time for the performance of all offensively noisy operations, between 10 in the Morning and 10 at Night—during which the industrious Housemaid may indulge her Arms in their full swing—and while she polishes her black-leaded grate to the lustre which is so lovely in the eyes of *"the Tidy,"* the TAT-TOO her brush strikes up against its sides may be performed without distressing the irritable ears of her Nervous Neighbours—to whom *undisturbed Repose is the most Vital Nourishment.*

Little Sweep Soot Ho is another dreadful disturber.—The shrill screaming of these poor boys, "making night hideous," (indeed at any time) at five or six o'clock in cold dark weather, is a most barbarous custom, and frequently disturbs a whole street before they rouse the drowsy sluggard who sent for him—his *Row dy Dow* when he reaches the top of the Chimney, and his progress down again, awaken the soundest sleepers, who often wish, that, instead of the Chimney,—he was smiting the skull of the Barbarian who set the poor Child to work at such an unseasonable hour.

The Editor's feelings are tremblingly alive on this subject.

    "Finis coronat opus."

However soundly he has slept during the early part of the night—if the finishing Nap in the morning is interrupted from continuing to its natural termination—his whole System is shook by it, and all that sleep has before done for him, is undone in an instant;—he gets up distracted and languid, and the only part of his head that is of any use to him, is the hole between his Nose and Chin.

The firm Health of those who live in the Country, arises not merely from breathing a purer Air,—but from quiet and regular habits, especially the enjoyment of plenty of undisturbed Repose,—this enables them to take Exercise, which gives them an Appetite, and by taking their food at less distant and more equally divided intervals—they receive a more regular supply of that salutary nourishment, which is necessary to restore the wear of the system, and support it in an uniform state of excitement,—equally exempt from the languor of inanition, and the fever of repletion.

Thus, the Animal Functions are performed with a perfection and regularity, the tranquillity of which, in the incessantly irregular habits of a Town-life, is continually interrupted,—some ridiculous Anxiety or other consumes the Animal Spirits, and the important process of Restoration is imperfectly performed.

Dyspeptic and Nervous disorders, and an inferior degree of both extensive and intensive Life[31] are the inevitable consequence, and are the lowest price for (what are called) *the Pleasures of Fashionable Society.*

Dr. Cadogan has told us (very truly) that Chronic diseases, (and we may add, most of those equivocal Disorders, which are continually teasing people, but are too insignificant to induce them to institute a medical process to remove them,) are caused by Indolence—Intemperance—and Vexation.

It is the fashion to refer all these Disorders to Debility—but Debility is no more than the effect of Indolence, Intemperance, and Vexation—the two first are under our own immediate control—and Temperance, Industry, and Activity, are the best remedies to prevent, or remove the Debility which reduces our means of resisting the third.

During *the Summer* of Life[32], *i. e.* the second period of it, (see page 34,) while we hope that every thing may come right, the Heart bounds with vigour, and the Vital flame burns too brightly to be much, or long subdued by vexation.

This originally least cause, soon becomes the greatest, and in *the Autumn* of our existence, when Experience has dissipated the theatric illusion with which Hope varnished the expectations of our earlier days, we begin to fear that every thing will go wrong.

> "The whips and scorns of Time,
> The oppressor's wrong, the proud man's contumely,
> The pangs of despis'd Love, the Law's delay,
> The insolence of office, and the spurns
> That patient merit of the unworthy takes."

The insatiable ruling passions of the second and third periods of Life,—Ambition and Avarice,—the loss of our first and best friends, our Parents,—regret for the past, and anxiety about the future, prevent the enjoyment of the present,—and are *the cause of those Nervous and Bilious Disorders*, which attack most of us at the commencement of the third period of Life—these *precursors of Palsy and Gout*, may generally be traced to Disappointments and Anxiety of mind[33]; and

People need not groan about the Insanities and Absurdities of others—it is surely quite sufficient to suffer for our own, of which most of us have plenty—we ought to endeavour to convert those of others, into causes of comfort and consolation, instead of fretting about them—if you receive rudeness in return for civility—and ingratitude for kindness, it may move your Pity—but should never excite your Anger—instead of murmuring at Heaven for having created such Crazy Creatures! be fervently thankful that you are not equally inconsistent and ridiculous—and Pray, that your own Mind, may not be afflicted with the like aberrations.

Indigestion[34], is the chief cause of perturbed Sleep, and often excites the imaginary presence of that troublesome Bedfellow *the Nightmare*. On this subject see *Peptic Precepts*

Some cannot Sleep if they eat any Supper—and certainly the lighter this meal is, the better—Others, need not put on their Night cap, if they do not first bribe their Stomachs to good behaviour by a certain quantity of Bread and Cheese and Beer, &c. &c., and go to Bed almost immediately after.

As to the wholesomeness of *a Solid Supper, per se,* we do not think it advisable,—but habit may have made it indispensable, and we know it is often the most comfortable Meal among the middle ranks of Society, who have as large a share of Health as any.

We caution *Bad sleepers* to beware how they indulge in the habit of exciting sleep, by taking any of the preparations of *Opium*—they are all injurious to the Stomach—and often inconvenient in their effects upon the Bowels:—

"REPOSE *by small fatigue is earned,* and Weariness can snore upon the flint, when nesty Sloth, finds a down pillow hard."

As there can be no good *Digestion* without diligent *Mastication,*—so there can be no sound *Sleep,* without sufficient *Exercise.*

The most inoffensive and agreeable Anodyne is to drink some good White Wine, or Mulled Wine, by way of a supplement to your Night cap.—One glass, taken when in Bed, immediately before lying down, is as effective as two or three if you sit up any time after.—(See *Tewahdiddle,* No. 467.)

Many people, if awoke during their first sleep, are unsettled all that night—and uncomfortable and nervous the following day.—The first sleep of those who eat Suppers, commonly terminates when the food passes from the

Stomach.—Invalids then awake, and sometimes remain so, in a Feverish state,—the Stomach feeling discontented from being unoccupied, and having nothing to play with:—a small crust of Bread, or a bit of Biscuit well chewed, accompanied or not, as Experience and Instinct will suggest, with a few mouthsful of Mutton or Beef Broth (No. 564), or Toast and Water (No. 463*), or single Grog[35], (*i. e.* one Brandy to nine Waters), will often restore its tranquillity, and catch Sleep again, which nothing invites so irresistibly, as introducing something to the Stomach,—that will entertain it, without fatiguing it.

We have heard persons say they have been much distressed by an intemperate craving for Food when they awoke out of their first sleep, and have not got to sleep soundly again after—and risen in the morning as tired as when they went to bed at night—but without any appetite for Breakfast —such will derive great benefit from the foregoing Advice.

A Broth (No. 564), *or Gruel* (No. 572) *Supper,* is perhaps the best for the Dyspeptic,—and those who have eaten and drank plentifully at Dinner.

THE BED ROOM should be in the quietest situation possible, as it were *"the Temple of Silence,"*—and, if possible, not less than 16 feet square—the height of this Apartment, *in which we pass almost half of our Time,* is in modern houses absurdly abridged, to increase that of the Drawing Room, which is often not occupied once in a month:—instead of living in the pleasant part of the House, where they might enjoy Light and Air, how often we find people squeezing themselves into "a nice snug Parlour," where Apollo cannot spy.

We do not recommend either *Curtains* or *Tester*, &c. to the BED, especially during the Summer;—by the help of these, those who might have the benefit of the free circulation of air in a large Room, very ingeniously contrive to reduce it to a small Closet:—*Chimney-Boards* and *Window-Curtains* are also inadmissible in a Bed Room; but Valetudinarians who are easily awoke, or very susceptible of Cold, will do wisely to avail themselves of well made *Double[36] Windows and Doors*, these exclude both Noise and Cold in a very considerable degree.

The best Bed is a well stuffed and well curled *Horsehair Mattress*, six inches thick at the Head, gradually diminishing to three at Feet, on this another Mattress five or six inches in thickness: these should be unpicked and exposed to the air, once every Year. An elastic Horsehair mattress, is incomparably the most pleasant, as well as the most wholesome Bed.

Bed Rooms should be thoroughly ventilated by leaving both the Window and the Door open every day when the weather is not cold or damp—during which the Bed should remain unmade, and the Clothes be taken off and spread out for an hour, at least, before the Bed is made again.

In very Hot Weather, the temperature becomes considerably cooler every minute after ten o'clock—between eight o'clock and twelve, the Thermometer often falls in Sultry weather—from ten to twenty degrees—and those who can sit up till twelve o'clock, will have the advantage of sleeping in an Atmosphere many degrees cooler, than those who go to bed at ten:—this is extremely important to Nervous Invalids—who however extremely they may suffer from heat, we cannot advise to sleep with the smallest part of the window open during the night—in such sultry days, the *Siesta* (see page 94,) will not only be a great support against the heat, but will help You to sit up to enjoy the advantage above stated.

A Fire in the Bed Room, is sometimes indispensable—but not as usually made—it is commonly lighted only just before bed-time, and prevents Sleep by the noise it makes, and the unaccustomed stimulus of its light.

Chimneys frequently smoke when a fire is first lighted, particularly in snowy and frosty weather; and an Invalid has to encounter not only the damp and cold of the Room—but has his Lungs irritated with the sulphureous puffs from the fresh lighted Fire.

A Fire should be lighted about three or four hours before, and so managed that it may burn entirely out half an hour before you go to Bed—then the air of the room will be comfortably warmed—and certainly more fit to receive an Invalid who has been sitting all day in a parlour as hot as an Oven,—than a damp chamber, that is as cold as a Well.

THE SIESTA.

The Power of *Position* and *Temperature* to alleviate the Paroxysms of many Chronic Disorders, has not received the consideration it deserves—a little attention to the variations of the Pulse, will soon point out the effect they produce on the Circulation, &c.—*extremes of Heat and Cold*, with respect to Food, Drink, and Air, are equally to be guarded against.

Old and Cold Stomachs—The Gouty—and those whose Digestive Faculties are Feeble—should never have any thing *Cold*[37], or *Old*, put into them—especially in Cold Weather.

Food must take the temperature of our Stomach, (which is probably not less than 120,) *before Digestion can commence.*

When the Stomach is feeble, *Cold Food* frequently produces Flatulence—Palpitation of the Heart, &c.—and all the other troublesome accompaniments of Indigestion.—The immediate remedy for these is Hot Brandy and Water, and the horizontal Posture.

Dyspeptic Invalids will find 75 a good temperature for their drink at Dinner, and 120 for Tea, &c.

Persons who are in a state of Debility from Age,—or other causes,—will derive much benefit from laying down, and seeking Repose whenever they feel fatigued, especially during (the first half-hour at least of) the business of Digestion—and will receive almost as much refreshment from half an hour's Sleep—as from Half a Pint of Wine.

The Restorative influence of the recumbent Posture, cannot be conceived—the increased energy it gives to the circulation, and to the organs of Digestion, can only be understood by those Invalids who have experienced the comforts of it.

The Siesta is not only advisable, but indispensable to those whose occupations oblige them to keep late hours.

ACTORS especially, whose profession is, of all others, the most fatiguing—and requires both the Mind and the Body to be in the most intense exertion between 10 and 12 o'clock at Night,—should avail themselves of the *Siesta*—which is the true source of Energy—half an hour's repose in the horizontal posture, is a most beneficial Restorative.

Good Beef Tea[38], (No. 563), with a little bit of slightly toasted Bread taken about nine o'clock—is a comforting restorative, which will support You through exertions that, without such assistance, are exhausting—and you go to bed fatigued—get up fevered, &c.

When Performers feel *Nervous*, &c.—and fear the circulation is below *Par*,—and too languid to afford the due excitement, half an hour before they sing, &c.—they will do wisely, to wind up their System, with a little "*Balsamum Vitæ*."—See "PEPTIC PRECEPTS."—Or tune their throats to the pitch of healthy vibration with a small glass of JOHNSON's[39] "*Witte Curacoa*," see (No. 474) and Index, a glass of Wine, or other stimulus.—

To "Wet your Whistle," is occasionally, as absolutely necessary, as "to rosin the Bow of a Violin."—See "Observations on Vocal Music," prefixed to the Opera of *Ivanhoe*.

ACTORS and SINGERS are continually assailed by a variety of circumstances extremely unfavourable to Health—especially from sitting up late at night—to counteract which, we recommend *the Siesta*, and plenty of Exercise in a pure Air.

When they feel *Nervous—Bilious*, &c. *i. e.* that their whole System is so deranged by fatigue and anxiety, that they cannot proceed effectively and comfortably,—they must give their Throats two or three days' rest—cleanse the Alimentary Canal with Peristaltic Persuaders—see Index—and corroborate the Organs of Digestion with the Tonic Tincture (No. 569), see Index.

Strong PEPPERMINT LOZENGES, made by SMITH, Fell Street, Wood Street, Cheapside, are very convenient portable Carminatives:—as soon as they are dissolved, their influence is felt from the beginning to the end of the Alimentary Canal—they dissipate Flatulence so immediately, that they well deserve the name of *Vegetable Ether*; and are recommended to SINGERS and PUBLIC SPEAKERS—as giving effective excitement to the Organs of Voice—

as a support against the distressing effects of Fasting too long—and to give energy to the Stomach between Meals.

THE POWER OF THE VOICE depends upon the vigorous state of the circulation supplying the Organs of Voice, with energy to execute the intentions of the Singer or Speaker—without which—the most accurate Ear and experienced Throat, will sometimes fail in producing the exact quality and quantity of Tone they intend.

That the VOICE is sometimes *too Flat*, or *too Sharp, &c.* is not a matter of astonishment—to those who really understand how arduous a task Singers have sometimes to perform;—it would only be wonderful if it was not—how is the Throat exempted from those collapses which occasionally render imperfect the action of every other fibre and function of our Body?

The *Dyspeptic*, who Tries the effect of Recumbency after Eating,—will soon be convinced that *Tristram Shandy* was right enough, when he said, that "both pain, and pleasure, are best supported in an horizontal posture."

"If after Dinner the Poppies of repletion shed their influence on thy Eyelids—indulge thou kind Nature's hint."—"A quiet slumber in a comfortable warm room, favoureth the operation of Digestion—and thou shalt rise, refreshed, and ready for the amusements of the Evening."

The *Semi-Siesta* is a pleasant position—(*i. e.* putting up the feet on a stool about eight inches high;) but catching a nap in a Chair is advisable only as a substitute when the Horizontal posture is not convenient—when you can, lie down on a Sofa—loosen all ligatures—and give your Bowels fair play.

These opinions,—which are the results of Personal experience—are exactly in unison with those of the following Medical Professors.

"From Eating comes Sleep—from Sleep Digestion."—SANCTORIUS, Sec. iv. Aph. 59.

"Perhaps one of the uses of Sleep, and of the horizontal posture during that period—may be to facilitate the introduction of Chyle into the Blood."—CRUICKSHANK *on the Absorbents*, p. 95.

"The Brute Creation invariably lay down and enjoy a state of rest, the moment their stomachs are filled. People who are feeble, digest their Dinner best, if they lie down and sleep as most Animals do, when their stomachs are full."—DARWIN's *Zoonomia*, vol. iv. p. 137.

"Dr. HARWOOD, Professor of Anatomy at Cambridge, took two pointers who were equally hungry, and fed them equally well,—*one* he suffered to follow the promptings of Instinct—curled himself round till he was comfortable—and went to sleep, as animals generally do after eating—the *other* was kept for about two hours in constant exercise. On his return home—the two Dogs were killed.—In the Stomach of the *one* who had been quiet and asleep, all the food was digested; in the Stomach of *the other*, that process was hardly begun."

"Quiet of Body and Mind for two hours after Dinner, is certainly useful to the Studious, the Delicate, and the Invalid."—ADAIR *on Diet*, p. 44.

"After Dinner, rest for three hours."—ABERNETHY's *Surgical Obs.* 8vo. 1817, p. 93.

"After Dinner sit a while."—*Eng. Prov.*

"If you have a strong propensity to Sleep after Dinner—indulge it, the process of Digestion goes on much better during Sleep, and I have always found an irresistible propensity to it—whenever Dyspeptic symptoms were considerable."—WALLER *on Incubus*, 1816, p. 109.

"Aged Men—and weak bodies, a short *Sleepe* after Dinner doth help to nourish."—LORD BACON's *Nat. Hist. Cent.* I. 57.

CLOTHES.

Of all the Customs of Clothing, the most extremely absurd is the usual arrangement of *Bed Clothes*, which in order as the chambermaid fancies to make the Bed look pretty in the Day time—are left long at the head, that they may cover the Pillows; when they are turned down, You have an intolerable load on your Lungs, and that part of the Body which is most exposed during the day—is smothered at night—with double the quantity of Clothes that any other part has.

Sleep is prevented by an unpleasant degree of either Heat or Cold; and in this ever-varying climate, where often "in one monstrous day all seasons mix," delicate Thermometrical persons will derive much comfort from keeping a Counterpane in reserve for an additional covering *in very Cold Weather:* when some extra clothing is as needful by Night,—as a great coat is by Day.

A Gentleman who has a mind to carry the adjustment of his Clothes to a nicety—may have the shelves of his Wardrobe numbered 30, 40, 50, 60, &c. and according to the degree of Cold pointed to by his Fahrenheit [40], he may wear a corresponding defence against it:—This mode of adjusting Dress according to the vicissitudes of the weather, &c. is as rational as the ordinary practice of regulating it by the Almanack, or the Fashion, which in this uncertain Climate and capricious Age—will as often lead us wrong, as right.

Leave off your Winter Clothes late in the Spring;—put them on early in the Autumn. By wearing your Winter Clothes during the first half dozen warm days—You get some fine perspirations—which are highly salutary in removing obstructions in the cutaneous pores, &c.

Delicate and Dyspeptic persons are often distressed by changing their Dress,—which must be as uniform as possible,—in thickness—in quality—and in form,—especially (Flannel, or indeed) whatever is worn next to the Skin.

The change of a thick Waistcoat for a thin one—or a long one for a shorter one—not putting on Winter garments soon enough, or leaving them off too soon,—will often excite a violent disorder in the Lungs—or Bowels, &c. and exasperate any constitutional complaint.

Those who wear *Flannel Waistcoats*, are recommended to have their new ones about the middle of November, with sleeves to them coming down to the wrist—the shortening these sleeves in the warm weather, is as effective an antidote against extreme Heat—as lengthening them, and closing the Cuff of the Coat, is against intense Cold.

Our COAT[41] should be made so large—that when buttoned we may be as easy as when it is unbuttoned, so that without any unpleasant increase of pressure on the Chest, &c. we can wear it closely buttoned up to the Chin—the power of doing this is a convenient provision against the sudden alternations from heat to cold—buttoning up this outer garment, will protect the delicate from many mischiefs which so often arise in this inconstant climate from the want of such a defence; and the additional warmth it produces will often cure slight Colds, &c.

Another way of accumulating Caloric, is to have two sets of button holes to the CUFF of the Coat, (especially of your Great Coat,) one of which will bring it quite close round the wrist.

When the Circulation is languid, and your *Feet are Cold*—wear worsted Stockings, have your Shoes well warmed—and when you take them from the Fire—put your Slippers[42] to it—that they may be warm and comfortable for you on your return home.

In Wet Weather wear Shoes with double upper-leathers—- two thin leathers will keep you much drier than one thick one, and are more pliable—the Currier's Dubbing is the best nourisher of Leather—and renders it as soft as satin, and impervious to Water.

The mean temperature of England is about 50 degrees of Fahrenheit—it sometimes rises 25 degrees above this, in the height of Summer,—falls about as much below, in the depth of Winter—and in Summer frequently varies from 20 to 30 degrees between Mid-day and Midnight.

The restoration, and the preservation of the Health, especially of those who have passed their FORTIETH *Year,—depends upon minute and unremitting* attentions to Food,—Clothes,—Exercise, &c. which taken singly may appear trifling—but combined, are of infinite importance.

"If you are careful of it, Glass will last as long as Iron." By a regular observance of a few salutary precepts, a delicate Constitution will last as long, and afford its Proprietor as many Amusements, as a Strong Body,—whose Mind takes but little care of it.

Invalids are advised to put on a Great Coat when they go out, and the temperature of the external air is not higher than 40. Some susceptible Constitutions require this additional clothing when the Thermometer falls below 50; especially at the commencement of the Cold weather.

A GREAT COAT must be kept in a Room where there is a Fire,—if it has been hung up in a cold damp Hall, as it often is, it will contribute about as much to your Calorification,—as if You wrapped a Wet Blanket about You.

Clothes should be warm enough to defend us from Cold[43],—and large[44] enough to let every movement be made with as much ease when they are on,—as when they are off.

Those whose employments are sedentary,—especially hard Students—who often neglect taking sufficient Exercise[45], suffer extremely from the pressure of tight *Waistbands—Garters, &c.* which are the cause of many of the mischiefs that arise from long sitting—during which they should be loosened.

Braces have been generally considered a great improvement in modern dress—because they render the pressure of the Waistband unnecessary, which when extremely close is certainly prejudicial—but we have always thought they have produced more inconvenience than they have removed—for if the inferior Viscera get thereby more freedom of action—the superior suffer for it—and, moreover, *Ruptures* are much more frequent—the Girdle which formerly prevented them being removed,—and, instead of that useful and partial horizontal pressure, in spite of the elastic springs which have been attached to the Braces, the whole body is grievously oppressed by the Vertical Bands.

FIRE.

As we advance in Age—the force of the circulation being lessened, the warmth of our Clothes and our coverings at night should be gradually increased. "After the age of 35, it may be better to exceed, rather than be deficient in clothing."—ADAIR's *Cautions*, p. 390.

Cold often kills the infirm and the aged, and is the proximate cause of most Palsies;—it is extremely desirable that Bed and Sitting Rooms for Winter occupation, should have a Southern aspect—when the Thermometer is below 30, the proper place for people beyond 60, is their own Fire-side:—many of the disorders and Deaths of persons at this period of Life—originate from irregularity in Diet, Temperature, &c. by Dining out, and frisking about, joining in Christmas Gambols, &c. in Cold weather.

The Art of making a room comfortably warm, does not consist merely in making a very large Fire in it—but depends as much on the keeping of cold air out—this is best done by *Double Windows*, see page 91, and double Doors,—at least take care that your Sashes fit close,—that the beads of the window frames are tight—stop the aperture between the skirting boards and the floor with putty—and list the Doors.

We suppose it almost needless to say that every room in the house should be thoroughly ventilated[47] by a current of fresh Air—at least once every day, when the weather is not very damp—or cold. By making a Fire accordingly —this may be done almost every Day in the Year.

If You leave the Door open for *Five* minutes—it will let in more cold air than your Fire can make warm in *Fifteen*—therefore, initiate your Domestics in these first principles of the *Economy of Caloric,*—and when the Weather is cold, caution them to keep Doors shut.

A regular Temperature may be preserved by a simple contrivance attached to a Thermometer, which will open an aperture to admit the external air—when the apartment is heated above the degree desired (*i. e.* about 60 for common constitutions,) and exclude it when it falls below it.

A Room, which is in constant occupation all day—may be occasionally *pumped* by moving the door backward and forward for several minutes.

We do not advise Invalids to indulge themselves in heating their rooms to a higher temperature[48] than from 60 to 65.—Those who have resided the best part of their Life in warm climates—will like the latter best. While we recommend the Aged and Infirm to be kept comfortably warm—they must at the same time cautiously avoid excess of heat.

When the Thermometer tells them that the external air is under 60,—whether it be in July, or in January,—those who are susceptible of Cold, must tell their Servants to keep a small fire—especially if the Weather be at the same time damp.

Those who, from caprice, or parsimony,—instead of obeying this comfortable and salutary precept, sit shivering and murmuring, and refuse to employ the Coal-merchant, as a substitute for the Sun—may soon spend in Physic, more than they have saved in Fuel.

By raising the temperature of my Room to about 65, taking a full dose of Epsom Salts, and a Broth Diet, and retiring to rest an hour sooner than usual, I have often very speedily got rid of *Colds*, &c.

The following *Plan of Lighting and managing a Fire*, has been attended with great comfort and convenience to myself, (particularly at the beginning and the end of winter, when a very small fire is sufficient), and I think considerable saving of coals.

Fill your Grate with fresh coals quite up to the upper bar but one, then lay in your faggot of wood in the usual manner, rather collected in a mass, than scattered, that a body of concentrated heat may be produced as soon as possible; over the faggot place the cinders of the preceding day—piled up as high as the grate will admit, and placed loosely in rather large fragments —in order that the draft may be free—a bit or two of fresh coal may be added to the cinders when once they are lighted, but no small coal must be thrown on at first, for the reason above stated:—when all is prepared, light the wood, when the cinders becoming in a short time thoroughly ignited—the gas rising from the coals below, which will now be effected by the heat, will take fire as it passes through them, leaving a very small portion of smoke to go up the Chimney.

The advantage of this mode of lighting a fire is, that small coal is better suited to the purpose than large—except a few pieces in front to keep the small from falling out of the Grate—it may be kept in reserve, to be put on afterwards if wanted. I have frequently known my fire lighted at 8 o'clock in the morning, continue burning till 11 at night, without any thing being done to it: when apparently quite out, on being stirred, you have in a few minutes a glowing fire: it will sometimes be necessary to loosen, or stir slightly the upper part of the fire if it begins to cake—but the lower part must not be touched, otherwise it will burn away too soon.

AIR.

Many Invalids are hurried into their Grave—by the indiscreet kindness of their friends forcing them from the comforts of Home—for the sake of Air more abounding with *Oxygen, i. e.* the vivifying part of the atmosphere:—that great benefit is received from what is *called* change of air is true enough—it is seldom considered that there is also a change in most of the other circumstances of the patient—many, of infinitely more importance, than that which derives all the credit of the Cure.

For instance, if a person living in a confined part of the City—neglecting exercise, harassed all day by the anxieties of Business, and sitting up late at Night, &c. be removed to the tranquillity of rural scenes, which invite him to be almost constantly taking Exercise in the open Air, and retiring to rest at an early hour—and thus, instead of being surrounded by irritations unfavourable to Health, enjoying all the *"jucunda oblivia vitæ"* which are favourable to it—such a Change will often do wonders, and sufficiently account for the miraculous cures attributed to—*Change of Air.*

Chemical Philosophers assert indeed—that a Gallon of the unsavoury Gas from Garlick Hill, gives as high a proportion of *Oxygen,* as the like quantity of the ethereal element of Primrose Hill:—this seems incredible, and must arise either from the imperfection of the *Eudiometer* giving erroneous results, or from the air being impregnated with matter unfriendly to Health, which the instruments employed to analyze it, have not the power of denoting:—let any one thread the mazes of a crowded city, and walk for the same space of time in a pleasant Country—the animal spirits will soon testify, which is the most exhilarating.

However, people certainly do live long, and enjoy Health, in situations apparently very unfavourable to Animal Life.

Our Omniscient Creator has given to our Lungs, the same faculty of extracting nutriment from various kinds of Air—as the Stomach has from various kinds of Aliment:—the Poor man who feeds on the coarsest food, is supported by it in as sound Health, as the Rich man who fares sumptuously every day.

Well then, in nine cases out of ten, to change the Atmosphere we have been long accustomed to, is as unadvisable as a change in the Food we have been used to—unless other circumstances make it so, than the mere change of Place.

The Opulent Invalid who has been long indulged with a Home arranged to his humour—must beware (especially during any exacerbation of his infirmity) of leaving it—it would be almost as desperate a procedure as to eject an Oyster from his Shells.

EXERCISE.

"By ceaseless action, all that is subsists,
Constant rotation of the unwearied wheel
That nature rides upon, maintains her health,
Her beauty, her fertility. She dreads an instant's pause,
And lives but while she moves."—COWPER'S *Task*.

"The wise, for Health on EXERCISE depend;
God never made his work for Man to mend."

The more luxuriously you live, the more Exercise[49] you require,—the "*Bon Vivant*" may depend upon the truth of the advice which Sir Charles Scarborough gave to the Duchess of Portsmouth, "You must Eat less,—or take more Exercise[50]—or take Physic,—or be Sick."

Exercise is the grand power to promote the Circulation through the capillary vessels, by which the constitution is preserved from obstructions,—Appetite increased, and Digestion improved in all its stages,—the due distribution of nourishment, invigorates the Nervous System, gives firmness and elasticity to the Muscles, and strength to every part of the System.

Exercise, to have its full effect, must be continued till we feel a sensible degree of *Perspiration*,—(which is the *Panacea for the prevention of Corpulence*)—see page 50—and should, at least once a-day, proceed to the borders of fatigue, but never pass them,—or we shall be weakened instead of strengthened.

Health depends upon perpetual Secretion and Absorption, and Exercise only can produce this.

After Exercise, take care to get cool gradually—when your Head perspires, rub it, and your Face, &c. dry with a cloth:—this is better for the Hair than the best "Bear's Grease," and will beautify the Complexion beyond "*La Cosmétique Royale*," or all the Red and White Olympian Dew that was ever imported.

One of the most important precepts for the preservation of Health, is to take care of *the Skin*[51].

In Winter, the surface of the Body, the Feet, &c. should be washed twice or thrice a Week, with water of the temperature of about 98, and wiped every Day with a wet towel;—*a Tepid Bath* of the like temperature once a fortnight will also conduce much to both health and comfort. Some advise that the surface of the Body be wiped every morning with a wet sponge, and rubbed dry after, with not too fine a cloth.

WINE.

"Le Vin est l'un des produits de la nature les plus difficiles à juger et à bien choisir: et les plus habiles gourmets sont souvent mis en défaut."—*Manuel du Sommelier*, Paris, 1817, p. 1.

Wine, especially Port, is generally twice spoiled—before it is considered fit to be drank!!!

The *Wine-Maker* spoils it first, by over-loading it with *Brandy* to make it keep.—

The *Wine-Drinker* keeps it till time has not only dissipated the superabundant spirit,—but even until the acetous fermentation begins to be evident,—this, it is the taste now to call *"Flavour,"*—and Wine is not liked, till it has lost so much of its exhilarating power, that you may drink a Pint of it, before receiving that degree of excitement,—which the Wine-drinker requires to make him Happy. We mean a legal PINT containing 16 ounces.

The measure of a BOTTLE OF WINE ought to be as definitive, as that of a POT OF PORTER:—is it not astonishing that the Legislature have not ordered *a Standard and Stamped Quart*, for the Wine-merchant—as they have a Pot for the Publican?

This would be equally as desirable to the respectable Wine-merchant,—as to the Public.

It would protect the former against the injurious competition of those who at present, by vending Wine in Bottles of inferior dimension, impose on the unwary purchaser under pretence of selling at a lower than the Market price.

The purchaser of a Dozen Bottles of Wine expects to receive Three Gallons of Wine.

Proportions of the Wine Gallon, according to the last London Pharmacopœia:—

Gallon.	Pints.	Fluid Ounces.	Drachms.	Minims or Drops.
1	= 8	= 128	= 1024	= 61,440

There are   32   ounces in a legal wine quart.
Multiply by   12   quarts in three gallons.

         ———

           384   ounces in ditto.

Measure the number of ounces your bottle holds—divide 384 by it, and the quotient will give you the number of such bottles required to contain three gallons of wine.

Some Bottles do not contain more than 26 ounces.

  26) 384 (14 Bottles, 1 Pint, and a Quarter.

    26

    ——

    124

    104

    ——

     20

            Or,

Multiply   26   *i. e.* the number of ounces
By   12   your bottle will contain.

                               ————

                     312   the number of ounces
                                 contained in your dozen
                                 bottles, which

Ought to hold   384   the number of ounces in
Subtract   312   Three Gallons.

                               ————

Divide by the number}   32) 72 (2 Quarts and half a Pint
of ounces in a Quart,}   64   short of measure.

—

8   ounces.

So, instead of THREE GALLONS—you have only *Two Gallons, one Quart, and a Pint and a half.*

The Quantity a Bottle will contain, may easily be accurately ascertained, by LYNES's *graduated Glass measure,* which holds half a pint, and is divided into ounces, &c.—*it is a convenient vessel to mix* GROG *in.*

A PIPE OF PORT contains, on the average, 138 Gallons, of which three must be allowed for Lees, &c.—This is enough for waste, if the Wine has been properly fined, and steadily bottled.

A BUTT OF SHERRY contains 130 gallons.
MADEIRA,   110 ditto.
Hogshead of CLARET,   55 ditto.

It is convenient for small Families to have part of their Wine in *Pint Bottles.*

That Wine is much best when quite fresh opened, is a fact it is needless to observe,—half a Pint of Wine (*i. e.* 8 ounces, *i. e.* 4 ordinary wine-glasses) is as much as most people (who have not spoiled their stomachs by intemperance) require.

The Rage for Superannuated Wine,—is one of the most *ridiculous Vulgar Errors of Modern Epicurism,*—"the Bee's Wing," "thick Crust[52] on the Bottle," "loss of strength, &c." which Wine-fanciers consider the Beauty of their tawny favourite, "fine Old Port,"—are forbidding manifestations of decomposition, and the departure of some of the best qualities of the Wine.

The Age[53] of maturity for exportation from Oporto, is said to be the second year after the Vintage, (probably sometimes not quite so long.)

Our Wine-merchants keep it in Wood from two to six years longer, according to its original strength, &c.—surely this must be long enough to do all that can be done by keeping it—what crude Wine it must be to require even this time to ameliorate it—the necessity for which, must arise either from some error in the original manufacture,—or a false taste, which does not relish it, till Time has changed its original characteristics.

Ordinary Port is a very uncleansed, fretful Wine—and experienced judges have assured us, that *the Best Port* is rather impoverished than improved, by being kept in Bottle longer than Two[54] Years, *i. e.* supposing it to have been previously from two to four years in the Cask in this Country,—observing, that all that the outrageous advocates for *"vin passé"*—really know about it, is, that SHERRY *is Yellow,*—and PORT *is Black,*—and that if they drink enough of either of them,—it will make them Drunk.

WHITE WINES, especially *Sherry* and *Madeira*, being more perfectly fermented, and thoroughly fined before they are bottled—if kept in a cellar of uniform temperature, are not so rapidly deteriorated by Age.

The Temperature of a Good Cellar is nearly the same throughout the year. *Double Doors* help to preserve this. It must be dry, and be kept as clean as possible.

The Art of preserving Wines, is to keep them from fretting, which is done by keeping them in the same degree of heat, and careful Corking[55]. "If persons wish to preserve the fine flavour of their Wines, they ought *on no account* to permit any Bacon, Cheese, Onions, Potatoes, or Cider, in their wine-cellars. Or, if there be any disagreeable stench in the Cellar, the wine will indubitably imbibe it; consequently, instead of being fragrant and charming to the nose and palate, it will be extremely disagreeable."—CARNELL *on Wine Making*, 8vo. 1814, p. 124. See also *Manuel du Sommelier, par A. Jullien*, Paris, 1817.

That MADEIRA (if properly matured before) improves in quality by being carried to the *East Indies* and back, by which Voyage it loses from 8 to 10 Gallons,—or to the *West*, by which about 5 are wasted[56],—however these round-about manœuvres may tickle the fancy of those folks who cannot relish any thing that is not far-fetched, dear-bought, and hard to be had, and to whom rarity is the *"sine qua non"* of recommendation—it is one of those inconvenient prejudices, from which common sense preserve us!

The Vulgar objection to *New Wine*—(by which we mean Wine that has been maturing in Wood two years in Portugal—two in England—and in Bottle more than twelve months), is, that its exhilarating qualities are too abundant, and intoxicate in too small a dose—those *"Bons Vivants,"* to whom "the Bottle, the Sun of the table," and who are not in the habit of crying to go home to Bed while they can see it shining,—require Wines weaker than those which are usually imported from Spain and Portugal,—however PORT and SHERRY may be easily reduced to the standard desired by the long-sitter,—"*paululum aceti acetosi,*" will give the Acid Goût,—"*aqua pura*" will subdue their Spirit "*ad libitum,*"—and produce *an imitation of the flavour acquired by Age, extempore*—and You can thus very easily make fine fruity nutritious new Wine,—as Light,—and as Old[57],—and as Poor, as you please—and fit it exactly to your customer's palate, whether "*Massa drinky for Drinky,—or drinky for Drunky Massa.*"

To ameliorate very new, or very old Wine—mix a bottle of the one with a bottle of the other—or to a bottle of very old Port add a glass or two of good new Claret—to very new, a glass of Sherry.

Of all our Senses,—*the Taste,* especially for Liquids, is the most sophisticated Slave of Habit—"De gustibus, non est disputandum."

The Astringent matter, and Alcohol—which render PORT WINE the prop of an Englishman's Heart—are intolerable to the palate of an Italian, or Frenchman.—But a Stomach which has been accustomed to be wound up by the double stimulus of Astringents, and Alcohol also,—will not be content with the latter only,—especially if that be in less quantity—as it is in the *Italian and French Wines*; which, therefore, for the generality of Englishmen, are insufficiently excitant.

He who has been in the habit of drinking PORTER at Dinner,—and PORT after —will feel uncomfortable with *Home-brewed Ale,* and *Claret.*

Mr. ACCUM, the chemist, analyzed for the Editor, some PORT and SHERRY of the finest quality—the PORT[58] yielded 20 per cent—and the SHERRY 19-25 per cent, of ALCOHOL of 825 specific gravity—*i. e.* the strongest Spirit of Wine that can be drawn, full double the strength of BRANDY, which seldom has 40 per Cent, and common GIN[59] not more than 30—or 25.

Some people have a notion that if they go to the Docks, they can purchase a Pipe of Wine for twenty pounds less, than they must pay to a regular Wine Merchant—and, moreover, have it *neat as imported*—as if all Wines of the same *Name,* were of the same Quality.

PORT *varies at Oporto in quality and price as much as* PORTER *does in London*—it is needless to say how difficult it is to obtain the best Beer at any price—it is quite as difficult to obtain the best Port Wine at Oporto, where the very superior wine is all bought up at a proportionately high price by the agents for the London Wine Merchants.

Brandies and Wines *vary in quality quite as much as they do in Price*: not less than twenty pounds per Pipe in the country where they are made.

The only way to obtain genuine wholesome liquor, is to apply to a respectable Wine Merchant—and beg of him to send you the best wine at the regular market price.

If you are particular about the Quality of what you buy—the less You ask about the price of it the better—if you are not, bargain as hard as you please.

The Editor buys his *Wines* of Messrs. Danvers and Clarke, No. 122, Upper Thames Street; his *Brandy and Liqueurs*[60] of Messrs. Johnson, in Pall Mall; and his *Spirits*, &c. of Mr. Rickards, Piccadilly.

A Moral and Physical Thermometer; or, a Scale of the Progress of Temperance and Intemperance, by J. C. Lettsom, M. D.

Liquors, *with their* Effects, *in their usual Order.*

TEMPERANCE

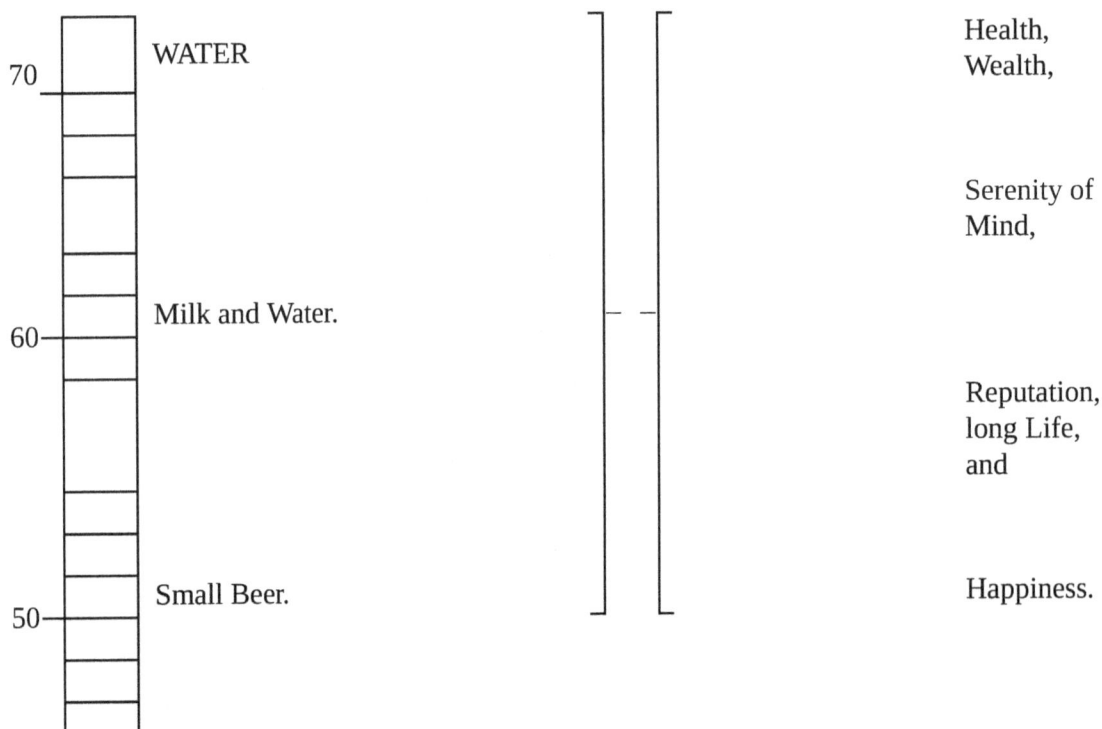

40 —	Cyder and Perry.	
30 —	Wine.	
	Porter.	
20 —		
	Strong Beer.	
10 —		

Cheerfulness,

Strength, and

Nourishment,
when taken

only at
Meals, and in

moderate
Quantities.

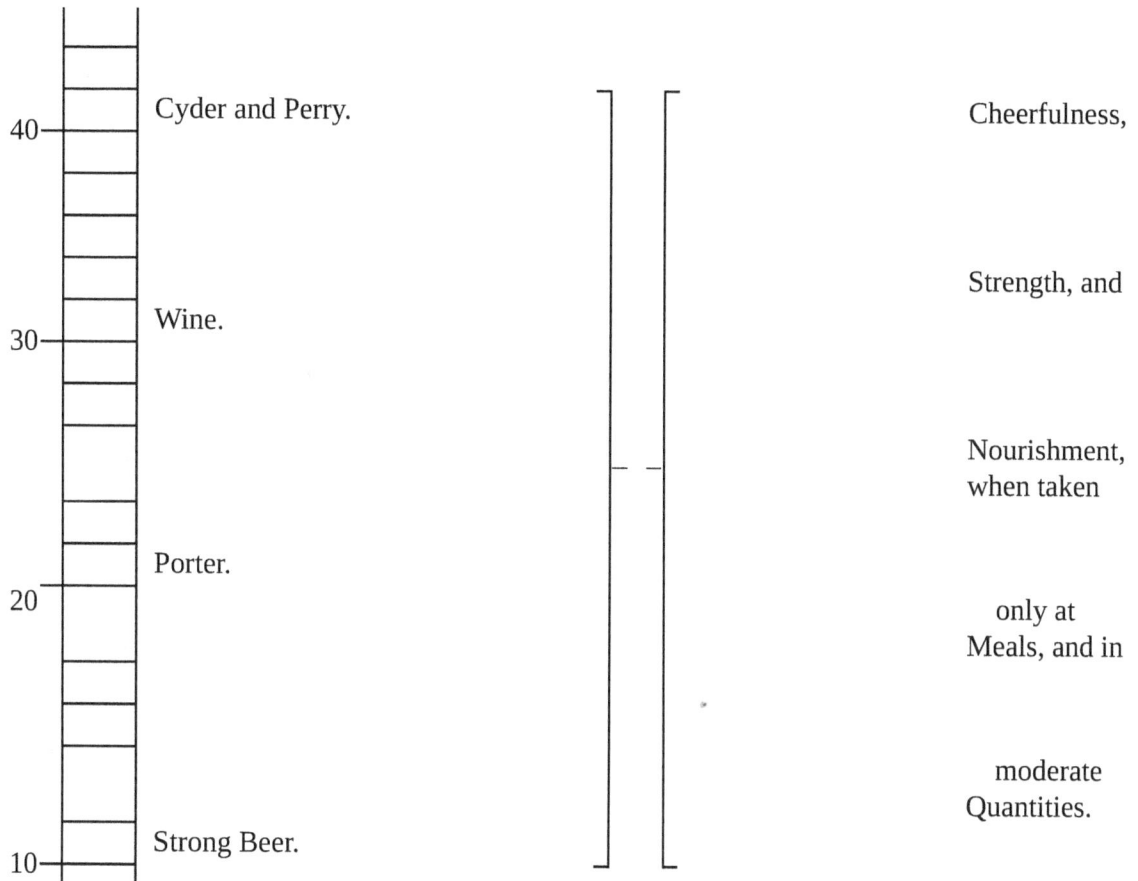

INTEMPERANCE

0 —		
	Punch.	
10 —		
	Toddy and Crank.	
20 —		
	{Grog, and	
30 —	{Brandy and	

VICES.	DISEASES.	PUNISHMENTS.
Idleness.	Sickness, Puking, and Tremors of the Hands in the Morning.	Debt.
Peevishness.		Black Eye.
Quarrelling.	Bloatedness.	
	Inflamed Eyes.	
Fighting.		Rags.

Scale	Liquors	Vices	Diseases	Punishments
	{Water.		Red Nose and Face.	
		Lying.	Sore and swelled Legs.	Hunger.
40	Flip and Shrub.	Swearing.	Jaundice.	Hospital.
	{Bitters infused	Obscenity.	Pains in the Limbs,	Poor-house.
	{in Spirits.		and burning in	
	{Usquebaugh.	Swindling.	the Palms of the	
50	{Hystericwater.		Hands, and Soles	Jail.
			of the Feet.	
	{Gin, Anniseed,	Perjury.	Dropsy.	Whipping.
	{Brandy,		Epilepsy.	
	{Rum, and	Burglary.	Melancholy.	The Hulks.
60	{Whisky in the		Madness.	
	{Morning.		Palsy.	Botany Bay.
		Murder.	Apoplexy.	
	{Do, during			
	{the Day and			
70	{Night.	Suicide.	DEATH.	GALLOWS.

Those who drink Wine[61], &c. for the purpose it was given, as a Cordial, to cheer the Circulation, when it falters from Fatigue, Age, or profuse Evacuations of any kind, "for the Stomach's sake," as St. Paul recommends it, and for our "often infirmities" as a medicine—will understand, that of all the ways of saving, to run any risk of buying inferior Wine, is the most ridiculously unwise Economy.

To *Ice Wine* is another very unprofitable and inconvenient custom—and not only deteriorates its flavour, but by rendering it dull in the mouth—people are induced to drink too much, as they are deprived of the advantage of knowing when they have got enough—for as soon as the Wine becomes warm in their Stomachs,—the dose they have taken merely to exhilarate them—makes them drunk.

The true Economy of Drinking,—is to excite as much Exhilaration as may be,—with as little Wine.

We deprecate the custom of *sitting for Hours after Dinner, and keeping the Stomach in an incessant state of irritation by sipping Wine,—nothing can be more prejudicial to Digestion*[62]—it is much better to mix Food and Drink —and to take them by alternate mouthsful.—See page 11.

Our "Vinum Britannicum"—good Home-brewed Beer—which has been very deservedly called *"Liquid Bread,"* is preferable to any other Beverage during Dinner or Supper—or *Port* or *Sherry* diluted with about three or four times their quantity of Toast and Water—(No. 463*): undiluted, these Wines are too strong to be drank during Dinner,—they act so powerfully on the feelings of the Stomach, that they dull the desire for solid Food, by producing the sensation of Restoration,—and the System, instead of receiving material to repair and strengthen it,—is merely stimulated during the action of the Vinous spirit.

However, the dull stimulus of Distention, is insufficient for some delicate Stomachs, which do absolutely require to be screwed up with a certain quantity of diffusible Stimulus[63],—without which, they cannot proceed effectively to the business of Digestion,—or indeed any other business—we do not recommend such, especially if they have passed the Meridian of Life, to attempt to entirely wean themselves of it—but advise them, *immediately after Dinner,* to drink as much as is necessary to excite that degree of action in their System, without which they are uncomfortable, and then to stop.—See Observations on *Siesta.*

Now-a-days, *Babies* are brought to table after Dinner by Children of larger growth—to drink Wine,—which has as bad an effect on their tender susceptible stomachs, as the like quantity of Alcohol would produce upon an Adult.

Wine has been called "the Milk of Old Age," so "Milk is the Wine of Youth." As Dr. Johnson observed, it is much easier to be abstinent than to be temperate—and no man should habitually take Wine as Food till he is past 30 years of age[64] at least;—happy is He who preserves this best of Cordials in reserve, and only takes it to support his Mind and Heart when distressed by anxiety and fatigue. That which may be a needful stimulus at

40 or 50, will inflame the Passions into madness at 20 or 30—and at an earlier period is absolute Poison.

Among other *innumerable Advantages which the Water-drinker enjoys*, remember he saves at least FIFTY GUINEAS per annum—which the Beer and Wine drinker wastes—as much to the detriment of his health, as the diminution of his Finances: moreover, nothing deteriorates the sense of Taste so soon as strong liquors—the *Water-drinker* enjoys an exquisite sensibility of Palate, and relish for plain food, that a Wine-drinker has no idea of.

Some people make it a rule to drink a certain number of Glasses of Wine during and after dinner, whether they are dry, or languid, or not—this is as ridiculous as it would be to eat a certain number of Mutton Chops whether you are hungry or not. The effect produced by Wine is seldom the same, even in the same person—and depends on the state of the animal spirits at the time—whether the stomach be full or empty, &c.

The more simply Life is supported, and the less Stimulus we use, the better —and Happy are the Young and Healthy who are wise enough to be convinced that Water is the best drink, and Salt the best sauce.

But in Invalids past the Meridian of Life, we believe as much mischief is going on when our Pulse hobbles along as if the Heart was too tired to carry on the Circulation, as can possibly be done to the constitution by taking such a portion of Wine as will remove the collapse—and excite the mainspring of Life to vibrate with healthful vigour.

The following is the Editor's plan of taking liquid food at Dinner,—when he cannot get Good Beer:—he has two wine glasses of Sherry, or one of Whiskey[65], or Brandy, (No. 471), and three-fourths of a pint of good Toast and Water, (No. 463), (which when Dyspeptic he has warmed to about Summer Heat, *i. e.* 75 of Fahrenheit,) and puts a wine-glass of Sherry, or half a glass of Whiskey, &c. into half a pint of the water, and the other glass of Sherry, or half glass of Whiskey, &c. into the remaining quarter pint— thus increasing the strength of the liquid towards the conclusion of Dinner, after which he drinks from two to four glasses of Port or Sherry—as Instinct suggests the state of the circulation requires—if it be very languid, a *Liqueur* glass of JOHNSON'S[66] *Witte Curaçoa*[67] is occasionally recommended as a renovating *Bonne Bouche*—about a quarter of an hour after dinner, he lies down on a Sofa, and sleeps for about half an hour—this has been his custom for the last twenty years—half an hour's horizontal posture is more restorative to him—than if he had sat up and drank three or four more glasses of wine.

As to *the Wholesomeness of various Wines*[68],—that depends on the integrity and skill of the Wine-maker,—and upon the peculiar state of the stomach of the Wine-drinker:—when my Stomach is not in Good Temper, —it generally desires to have *Red Wine,*—but when in best Health,— nothing affronts it more than to put *Port* into it—and one of the first symptoms of its coming into adjustment, is a wish for *White Wine.*

One of the chief causes of that derangement of the Stomach, which delicate and aged persons so constantly complain of after *Dining out*—is the drinking of Wines, &c. which they are unused to.

White, deserve to be preferred to *Red Wines,*—because the latter being harder pressed, and subjected to a stronger fermentation to extract the colouring matter from the husks of the Grape, are more loaded with feculence.

Of RED WINES, *Claret* is the best; and it is to be lamented, that the Duty imposed upon it is so great, that to moderate fortunes it amounts to a prohibition—when we make this observation, we do not mean to impeach the prudence which has induced those who no doubt best understand the subject,—to determine that political necessity imperatively decrees that the delightful and salubrious wines of France—must be taxed twice as high as the coarse unwholesome wines of Portugal.

Of the *White* Wines, we believe that *Sherry* is the most easy—and *Madeira* the most difficult to obtain genuine—most of the SWEET Wines are as artificially compounded, as the Beers of this country; the addition of Capillaire to Port wine, makes what is commonly called *Tent. Mountain, Calcavella, &c.* are made up in the same manner.

For further Illustrations of this subject, see ACCUM *on Adulterations*, 2d Edition, 12mo. 1820.

An Inquiry into the Effects of Fermented Liquors, by a Water-drinker, 2d Edit. 1818.

SANDFORD's *Remarks on Wine*. Worcester, 1799.

LETTSOM, *on the Effects of Hard Drinking*.

TROTTER, *on Drunkenness*, 1804.

ACCUM's *Art of making English Wine*, 1820.

CARNELL, *on Family Wine Making*, 1814.

ACCUM, *on Brewing*, 1820.

RAWLINSON, *on Brewing in Small Quantities,*—printed for Johnson, 1807, price 1s.; *and Home Brewed Ale*, printed for Robinson, 1804, price 2s.

Facts Proving Water the best Beverage. Printed by Smeeton, in St. Martin's Lane.

Manuel de Sommelier, par A. JULLIEN, Paris, 1817.

PEPTIC PRECEPTS.

"Suaviter in modo, sed fortiter in re."

Not one Constitution in a thousand, is so happily constructed or is constantly in such perfect adjustment, that the operations of the Abdominal Viscera (on which every other movement of the system depends) proceed with healthful regularity.

The following hints will point out to the Reader, how to employ Art to afford that assistance to Nature, which in Indisposition and Age, is so often required, and will teach him to counteract in the most prompt and agreeable manner—the effects of those accidental deviations from strict Temperance, —which sometimes overcome the most abstemious philosopher—when the seducing charms of Conviviality tempt him to forego the prudent maxims of his cooler moments.

They will help those who have delicate Constitutions, to obtain their fair share of Health and Strength,—and instruct the Weak, so to economize the powers they have, that they may enjoy Life as well as the Strong.

To humour that desire for the marvellous, which is so universal in medical (as well as in other) matters,—the makers of *Aperient Pills* generally select the most DRASTIC PURGATIVES, which operating considerably in a dose of a few grains, excite admiration in the Patient, and faith in their powers, in proportion as a small dose produces a great effect,—who seldom considers how irritating such materials must be,—and consequently how injurious to a Stomach in a state of Debility, and perhaps deranged by indulging Appetite beyond the bounds of moderation.

INDIGESTION will sometimes overtake the most experienced Epicure;—when the gustatory nerves are in good humour, Hunger and Savoury Viands will sometimes seduce the Tongue of a *"Grand Gourmand"* to betray the interest of his Stomach[69] in spite of his Brains.

On such an unfortunate occasion,—whether the intestinal commotion be excited by having eaten too much, or too strong food—lie down—have your Tea early after Dinner—and drink it warm.

This is a hint to help the Invalid, whose digestion is so delicate, that it is sometimes disordered by a Meal of the strictest Temperance. If the anxiety, &c. about the Stomach does not speedily abate, apply the *"Stomach Warmer."* This valuable companion to Aged and Gouty Subjects, may be procured at No. 58, Haymarket.

A certain degree of Heat is absolutely necessary to excite and support a regular process of Digestion;—when the Circulation is languid, and the food difficult of solution, in Aged persons and Invalids,—*External Heat* will considerably assist Concoction, and the application of this calificient concave will enable the Digestive organs to overcome refractory materials, —and convert them into laudable Chyle.

Unless the Constitution is so confoundedly debilitated, that the Circulation cannot run alone—*Abstinence*[70] is the easiest—cheapest—and best cure for the disorders which arise from *Indigestion* or *Intemperance.* I do not mean what Celsus calls the first degree of it, "when the sick man takes nothing," but the second, "when he takes nothing but what he ought."

The Chylopoietic organs are uncomfortable when entirely unoccupied,— when the Stomach is too tired to work, and too weak to be employed on actual service,—it desires something to be introduced to it, that will entertain it till it recovers its energy.

After INTEMPERATE FEASTING one day, let the food of the following day be Liquid, or of such materials as are easy of solution.

Various expedients have been recommended for preventing and relieving the disorders arising from too copious libations of "the Regal purple Stream."

When a good fellow has been sacrificing rather too liberally at the shrine of the Jolly God, the best remedy to help the Stomach to get rid of its burthen, is to take for Supper some GRUEL, (No. 572, *see Index,*) with half an ounce of Butter, and a teaspoonful of *Epsom Salt* in it; or two or three *Peristaltic Persuaders,*—which some Gastropholists take as a provocative to appetite, about an hour before Dinner.

Some persons take as a *"sequitur"* a drachm of *Carbonate of Soda.*

Others a teaspoonful of *Calcined Magnesia:*—when immediate relief is required, never administer this uncertain medicine, which, if the Stomach has no Acid ready to dissolve it,—will remain inert; it must be taken, only when *Heart-burn* and symptoms of Acidity are manifest.

As a *Finale* to the day of the Feast, or the *Overture* of the day after, take (No. 481*,) or two drachms of *Epsom Salt* in half a pint of *Beef Tea,*—or some *Tincture of Rhubarb* in hot water,—the first thing to be done, is to endeavour to get rid of the offending material.

A Breakfast of *Beef Tea*[71] (No. 563,) is an excellent Restorative;—when *the Languor following Hard Drinking* is very distressing, indulge in the horizontal posture; (see *Siesta,* p. 94;) nothing relieves it so effectually, or so soon cheers the Circulation, and sets all right;—get an early Luncheon of restorative Broth or Soup.

HARD DRINKING *is doubly debilitating, when pursued beyond the usual hour of retiring to Rest.*

Those devotees to the Bottle, who never suffer the orgies of Bacchus to encroach on the time which Nature demands for Sleep,—escape with impunity, many of the evils which soon—and irreparably—impair the Health of the Midnight reveller.

A facetious observer of the inordinate degree in which some people will indulge their Palate, to the gratification of which they sacrifice all their other senses,—recommends such to have their Soup seasoned with a tasteless purgative, as the Food of insane persons sometimes is, and so prepare their bowels for the hard work they are going to give them!!

To let the Stomach have a holiday occasionally—*i. e.* a Liquid diet, of Broth and Vegetable Soup, is one of the most agreeable and most wholesome ways of restoring its Tone.

If your Appetite[72] *be languid,* take additional Exercise in a pure open Air,— or Dine half an hour later than usual, and so give time for the Gastric Juices to assemble in full force;—or dine upon Fish—or *Chinese Soup, i. e.* Tea.

If these simple means are ineffectual,—the next step, is to produce energetic vibration in the Alimentary tube, without exciting inordinate action, or debilitating depletion; and to empty the Bowels, without irritating them.

Sometimes *when the languor occasioned by Dyspepsia, &c. is extreme*, the Torpor of the System becomes so tremendous—that no Stimulus will help it, and the Heart feels as if it was tired of beating—a moderate dose of a quickly operating Aperient, *i. e.* half an ounce of Tincture of Rhubarb, and two drachms of Epsom Salts in a tumbler of hot water—will speedily restore its wonted energy.

THE STOMACH is the centre of Sympathy;—if the most minute fibre of the human frame be hurt, intelligence of the injury instantaneously arrives;—and the Stomach is disturbed, in proportion to the importance of the Member, and the degree in which it is offended.

If either the Body or the Mind be fatigued,—the Stomach invariably sympathizes;—if the most robust do any thing too much, the Stomach is soon affronted,—and does too little:—unless this mainspring of Health be in perfect adjustment, the machinery of life will vibrate with languor;—especially those parts which are naturally weak, or have been injured by Accidents, &c. Constipation is increased in costive habits—and Diarrhœa in such as are subject thereto—and all Chronic complaints are exasperated, especially in persons past the age of 35 years.

Of the various helps to Science, none perhaps more rapidly facilitate the acquirement of knowledge, than analogical reasoning; or illustrating an Art we are ignorant of, by one we are acquainted with.

THE HUMAN FRAME may be compared to a Watch, of which the Heart is the Mainspring—the Stomach the regulator,—and what we put into it, the Key by which the machine is wound up;—*according to the quantity,—quality,—and proper digestion of what we Eat*[73] *and Drink, will be the pace of the Pulse, and the action of the System in general:*—when we observe a due proportion between the quantum of Exercise and that of Excitement, all goes well.—If the machine be disordered, the same expedients are employed for its re-adjustment, as are used by the Watch-maker; it must be carefully cleaned, and judiciously oiled.

Eating *Salads* after Dinner,—and chilling the Stomach, and checking the process of digestion by swilling cold *Soda Water*—we hold to be other Vulgar Errors.

It is your superfluous SECOND COURSES,—and ridiculous variety of Wines,—Liqueurs,—Ices, Desserts, &c.—which (are served up more to gratify the pride of the Host, than the appetite of the Guests that) *overcome the Stomach, and paralyze Digestion,* and seduce "Children of larger Growth" to sacrifice the health and comfort of several days—for the Baby-pleasure of tickling their tongue for a few minutes, with Trifles and Custards!!

Most of those who have written on what—by a strange perversion of language—are most non-naturally termed the non-naturals,—have merely laid before the Public a nonsensical register of the peculiarities of their own Palate, and the idiosyncrasies of their own Constitution[74].

Some omnivorous Cormorants have such an ever-craving Appetite, that they are raging with hunger as soon as they open their Eyes,—and bolt half a dozen hard Eggs before they are well awake;—Others are so perfectly restored by that "chief nourisher in Life's feast," Balmy Sleep, that they do not think about Eating,—till they have been up and actively employed for several hours.

The strong Food, which the strong action of strong bodies requires—would soon destroy weak ones,—if the latter attempt to follow the example of the former,—instead of feeling invigorated, their Stomachs will be as oppressed, as a Porter is with a load that is too heavy for him,—and, under the idea of swallowing what are called strengthening nourishing things,—will very soon make themselves ready for the Undertaker.

Some people seem to think, that the more plentifully they stuff themselves, the better they must thrive, and the stronger they must grow.

It is not the quantity that we swallow,—but that which is properly digested, which nourishes us.

A Moderate Meal well digested, renders the body vigorous,—glutting it with superfluity, (which is only turned into excrement instead of aliment, and if not speedily evacuated,) not only oppresses the System, but produces all sorts of Disorders.

Some are continually inviting *Indigestion*,—by eating *Water-cresses*, or other undressed Vegetables[75], "to sweeten their Blood,"—or *Oysters* "to enrich it."—Others fancy their Dinner cannot digest till they have closed the orifice of their Stomachs with a certain portion of *Cheese*,—if the preceding Dinner has been a light one, a little bit of Cheese after it may not do much harm, but its character for encouraging concoction is undeserved, —there is not a more absurd Vulgar Error, than the often quoted proverb, that

"Cheese is a surly Elf,

Digesting all things, but itself."

A Third never eats Goose, &c. without remembering that *Brandy* or *Cayenne* is the Latin for it.

A much less portion of Stimulus is necessary after a hearty meal of califactive materials, such as good Beef or Mutton—than after a *maigre* Dinner of Fish, &c.

Another *Vulgar Error* in the school of Good Living, is, that *"Good eating* requires *Good drinking."*—*Good* eating generally implies *high* seasoned Viands,—the savoury Herbs, and stimulating Spices with which these *Haut-Gouts* are sprinkled and stuffed, &c. are sufficient to encourage the digestive faculties to work *"con amore"* without any *"douceur"* of Vinous irrigation,—but many persons make it a rule, after eating Pig, &c. to take a glass of *Liqueur*, or *Eau de Vie*, &c.—or, as when used in this manner, it would be as properly called, *"eau de mort."*

INDIGESTION, or, to use the term of the day, A BILIOUS ATTACK,—*as often arises from over-exertion, or* ANXIETY OF MIND,—as from refractory Food; it frequently produces FLATULENCE[76], and flatulence produces *Palpitation of the Heart*; which is most difficult to stop, when it comes on about an hour or two after a Meal;—the Stomach seems incapable of proceeding in its business, from being over-distended with wind, which pressing on the Heart and larger vessels, obstructs the Circulation:—as soon as this flatulence is dispelled, all goes well again:—inflating the Lungs to the utmost, *i. e.* taking in as much breath as you can, and holding it as long as you can, will sometimes act as a counterbalance, and produce relief.

This is the first thing to do when this distressing Spasm attacks you,—if it is not immediately checked; take a strong *Peppermint*, or *Ginger Lozenge*, (see page 99,) sit, —or if possible lie down and loosen all ligatures; the horizontal posture and perfect quiet are grand Panaceas in this disorder;—if these do not soon settle it, drink some stimulus: sometimes a teacupful of *Hot water*, with a teaspoonful of common salt in it, will suffice,—or a couple of glasses of *Wine*,—or one of *Brandy* in one of hot water: either of these will generally soon restore sufficient energy to the Stomach, to enable it to expel the enemy that offends it, and set the circulation to work freely again.—If these means are not immediately efficacious, take half an ounce of *Tincture of Rhubarb* in a quarter pint of hot water,—or three or four *Peristaltic Persuaders*, with half a pint of hot water.

If this complaint comes on when the Bowels are costive,—they must be put into motion as speedily as possible, by some of the means recommended in the following pages.

It will sometimes come on during the collapsed state of the system, from FASTING TOO LONG.

Those who take no Food between an early BREAKFAST—*and a late* DINNER,—for fear, as they term it, of spoiling the latter meal,—generally complain of *Flatulence,—Languor, Lowness of Spirits,* &c. (and those who are troubled by a *Cough,* have often a paroxysm of it,) for the hour or more before Dinner;—and *Heartburn,* &c. after it:—the former arising from fasting too long, the latter from indulging an Appetite so over excited, that a Baron of Beef, a Pail of Port Wine, and a Tubful of Tea, will hardly satisfy it.

The languor of *Inanition,* and the fever of *Repletion,* may be easily avoided by eating a LUNCHEON,—solid and nutritive, in proportion as the DINNER is protracted, and the activity of the Exercise to be taken in the mean-time.

The oftener you eat, the less ought to be eaten at a time; and the less you eat at a time, the oftener you ought to eat:—*a weak Stomach* has a much better chance of digesting two light meals, than one heavy one.

The Stomach should be allowed time to empty itself, before we fill it again.

There is not only a considerable difference in the digestibility of various Foods,—but also of the time required by different Stomachs to digest them —the sign of which, is the return of Appetite.

The digestion of Aliment is perfect, and quickly performed, in proportion to the keenness of our Appetite at the time of taking it—more or less perfect Mastication—and the vigorous state of the organs of Digestion,—as a general rule, *the interval of Fasting* should seldom be less than three, nor more than five hours[77],—Digestion being generally completed within that time.

The Fashion of A.D. 1820 has introduced a much longer fast ("a windy recreation," as father Paul assures the lay brother) than even the elasticity of robust Health can endure, without distressing the adjustment of the System, —and creating such an over-excited appetite, that the Stomach does not feel it has had enough,—till it finds that it has been crammed too much[78].

> "When Hunger[79] calls, obey, nor often wait
> Till hunger sharpen to corrosive pain;
> For the keen appetite will feast beyond
> What nature well can bear."

This important truth—we would most strongly press on the consideration of Those who attend our COURTS OF LAW, and PARLIAMENT.

Many industrious Professional men, in order to add a few pounds to their Income—in a few years are quite worn out—from their digestive faculties being continually disordered and fretted for want of *regular* supplies of *Food*; and sufficient *Sleep*.

An Egg boiled in the shell for five minutes, or *Les Tablettes de Bouillon* (No. 252), and a bit of Bread, is a convenient provision against the former —*the Siesta* (see page 94) is the best Antidote for the latter.

The sensation of *Hunger* arises from the Gastric juices acting upon the coats of the Stomach—how injurious it must be to fast so long, that by neglecting to supply it with some alimentary substance which this fluid was formed to dissolve,—the Stomach becomes in danger of being digested itself!!!

Those who feel a gnawing, as they call it, in their Stomach, should not wait till the stated hour of dinner, but eat a little forthwith, that the Stomach may have something to work upon.

By *too long Fasting*, Wind accumulates in the Stomach, especially of those who have passed the meridian of Life—and produces a distressing Flatulence—Languor—Faintness—Giddiness—Palpitation of the Heart, &c.

If the Morning has been occupied by anxiety in Business,—or the Mind or Body is fatigued by over-exertion—these symptoms will sometimes come on about an hour or two before the usual time of Dining,—well masticating a bit of Biscuit, and letting a strong Peppermint Lozenge (see page 99) dissolve in the mouth as soon as you feel the first symptoms of Flatulence, —will often pacify the Stomach, and prevent the increase of these complaints.

Dr. Whytt, whose observations on *Nervous Disorders*, (like this work), are valuable, inasmuch as they are the authentic narrative of his own Experience—says, page 344, "When my Stomach has been weak, after I have been indisposed, I have often found myself much better for a glass of Claret and a bit of bread, an hour or more before Dinner, and I have ordered it in the same way to others, and again in the evening, an hour or more before Supper, with advantage."

There is no doubt of the propriety of Dr. W.'s prescription, the Editor's own feelings bear witness to it. For those who are just recovering from Diseases which have left them in a state of great Debility, a glass of Wine and a bit of Bread,—or a cup of good *Beef Tea*, (see page 96) are perhaps as good Tonics as any,—they not only remove Languor, but at the same time furnish Nutriment.

We have known weak Stomachs, when kept fasting beyond the time they expected,—become so exhausted—they would refuse to receive any solid Food,—until restored to good temper,—and wound up by some Wine, or other stimulus—as Instinct proposed.

Feeble Persons, who are subject to such sudden attacks, should always travel armed with a *Pocket Pistol* charged with a couple of glasses of White Wine, or, "*Veritable Eau de Vie*,"—a Biscuit, and some strong Peppermint or Ginger Lozenges, or see "*Tablettes de Bouillon*" (No. 252):—when their Stomach is uneasy from emptiness, &c. these crutches will support the Circulation,—and considerably diminish, and sometimes entirely prevent the distressing effects which Invalids suffer from too long a Fast[80].

What a contrast there is between the materials of the morning meal A.D. 1550, when Queen Elizabeth's Maids of Honour began the day with a *Round of Beef*,—or a *Red Herring*, and a *flaggon of Ale*—and in 1821, when the Sportsman, and even the day-Labourer, breakfast on what Cooks call "*Chinese Soup*," i. e. Tea.

Swift has jocosely observed, such is the extent of modern Epicurism, that "*the World*[81] *must be encompassed—before a Washerwoman can sit down to Breakfast,*" *i. e.* by a voyage to the East for Tea, and to the West for Sugar.

In THE NORTHUMBERLAND HOUSEHOLD BOOK for 1512, we are informed that "*a Thousand Pounds* was the sum annually expended in Housekeeping,— this *maintained* 166 *Persons,*—and the Wheat was then 5*s*. 8*d*. per quarter.

"The Family rose at six in the morning,—my Lord and my Lady had set on their Table for BREAKFAST, *at Seven o'clock* in the morning,

> A quart of Beer,
> A quart of Wine,
> Two pieces of Salt Fish,
> Half a dozen Red Herrings,
> Four White ones, and
> A Dish of Sprats!!!

"*They* DINED *at Ten*—SUPPED *at Four* in the afternoon,—The Gates were all shut at nine, and no further ingress or egress permitted."—See pages 314 and 318.

But now, A.D. 1821,

> "The Gentleman who dines the latest
> Is, in our Street, esteemed the greatest:
> But surely greater than them all,
> Is he who never Dines[82] at all."

DINNERS at *Night,*

AND

SUPPERS in the *Morning,*

A few Cautionary Hints to Modern Fashionables.—

> "The Ancients did delight, forsooth,
> To sport in allegoric Truth;
> Apollo, as we long have read since,
> Was God of Music, and of Med'cines.
> *In Prose,* APOLLO is the Sun,

And when he has his course begun,
The allegory then implies
'Tis Time for wise men to arise;
For ancient sages all commend
The morning, as the Muses friend;
But modern Wits are seldom able
To sift the moral of this fable;—
But give to Sleep's oblivious power
The treasures of the morning hour,
And leave reluctant, and with Pain,
With feeble nerve, and muddy Brain,
Their favorite couches late at noon,
And quit them then perhaps too soon,
Mistaking by a sunblind sight
The Night for Day—and Day for Night.
Quitting their healthful guide Apollo,
What fatal follies do they follow!
Dinners at night—and in the Morn
Suppers, serv'd up as if in scorn
Of Nature's wholesome regulations,
Both in their Viands and Potations.
Besides, Apollo is M. D.
As all Mythologists agree,
And skill'd in Herbs and all their virtues,
As well as Ayton is, or Curtis.
No doubt his excellence would stoop
To dictate a Receipt for *Soup*,
Show as much skill in dressing *Salad*,
As in composing of a *Ballad*,
'Twixt Health and Riot draw a line,
And teach us How—and When—to dine.
The Stomach, that great Organ, soon,
If overcharg'd, is out of tune,
Blown up with Wind that sore annoys
The Ear with most unhallow'd noise!!
Now all these Sorrows and Diseases
A man may fly from if he pleases;

For rising early will restore
His powers to what they were before,
Teach him to Dine at Nature's call,
And to Sup lightly, if at all;
Teach him each morning to preserve
The active brain, and steady nerve;
Provide him with a share of Health
For the pursuit of fame, or wealth;
And leave the folly of *Night Dinners*
To Fools and Dandies, and Old Sinners!!!"

That distressing interruption of the Circulation, which is called "NIGHTMARE," "Globus Hystericus," "Spasms," "Cramp," or "Gout," in the Stomach, with which few who have passed the Meridian of Life[83], are so fortunate as not to be too well acquainted, we believe to arise from the same causes—which in the day produce Palpitation of the Heart.

The Editor is now in his forty-third year, and has been from his youth occasionally afflicted with both these disorders; sometimes without being able to imagine what has produced them:—sometimes he has not been attacked with either of these complaints for many months; they have then seized him for a week or more,—and as unaccountably ceased.

THE NIGHTMARE has generally come on about three o'clock in the morning, —at the termination of the first, or rather at the commencement of the second sleep;—quite as often when he has taken only a liquid or very light supper,—as when he has eaten some solid food, and gone to bed soon after; —and most frequently after he has Dined[84] out: not from the quantity, but the quality of the food and drink he has taken, the change of the time of taking it. The fatigue attending his performance of Amphytrion at his own table, has also occasionally produced it.

It appears to be occasioned by want of Action in the System, being generally preceded by Languor—(which, if not removed, may proceed to produce—*Palsy*—or *Death*,) caused either by depression of the power of the Heart by anxiety,—obstruction of the peristaltic motion by the oppression of indigestible matter,—or interruption of the performance of the Restorative Process.

It is certainly not to be prevented by Abstinence, for during the time that the Editor was trying the effect of a spare diet, he was most frequently afflicted with it.—See *Obs.* on SLEEP, &c. It is only to be relieved by Stimulants, and in an extreme case—by quickly acting Aperients, &c. See following pages.

Some persons are peculiarly subject to it when they lie on their back,—others if on their left side:—when the Editor has any disposition to this malady, it is certainly exasperated if he lays upon his right side,—especially during the first part of the Night,—it is a good Custom to lay one half of the Night on one side, and the other half on the other.

When this appalling pause of the Circulation takes place—he wakes, with the idea that another minute of such suspended action will terminate his Existence:—his first recourse is to force the action of the Lungs by breathing as quick and as deep as possible.—He feels very languid,—and to prevent a return of the fit, drinks a couple of glasses of *White Wine,*—or half a wine-glass of *Brandy,* in a wine-glass of *Peppermint Water.*

Sometimes the Disorder does not terminate with one paroxysm, but recurs as soon as Sleep returns:—when this is the case, get half a tumbler of Hot Water, add to it a wine-glass of *Peppermint Water,* and half that quantity of *Tincture of Rhubarb,* or fifty drops of *Sal Volatile,* or both.

The symptom of security from a repetition of the Fit, is a vermicular sensation, betokening that the peristaltic motion, and the Circulation is restored to its regular pace again.

His belief that many sudden and unaccountable Deaths in the night have arisen from Invalids not knowing how to manage this Disorder, induces the Editor to relate his own personal experience concerning it—and the Remedies which he has found effectual to remove it.

"Non ignara mali, miseris succurrere disco."

The case is very similar to what Dr. WHYTT relates of himself, in his *Observations on Nervous, Hysteric, and Hypochondriac Disorders,* 8vo. 1767[85]; by which, Dr. CULLEN, in p. 10 of his *Clinical Lectures,* says, "he has done more than all his predecessors."

Mr. WALLER has written a very sensible Essay on the *Nightmare*—those who are much afflicted with it, cannot lay out 3*s.* 6*d.* better, than in buying his book—12mo. 1816. He says, "it most frequently proceeds from acidity in the Stomach, and recommends *Carbonate of Soda,* to be taken in the Beer you Drink at dinner." He tells us "he derived his information, as to the cause, and cure of this distressing disorder, from a personal acquaintance with it for many years."

How devoutly it is to be wished that all Authors would follow good old SYDENHAM and Mr. WALLER'S example,—and give us a register of the progress of those chronic complaints which they have themselves been afflicted with, and the regimen, &c. which they have found most effectual to alleviate and cure them;—and, instead of what they think,—write only what they know,—as the pains-taking SANCTORIUS—SPALLANZANI—BRYAN ROBINSON,—and the persevering and minutely accurately observing Dr. STARK have in their *Dietetical Experiments.*

Dr. WHYTT has immortalized himself by the candid relation of his own infirmities, and his circumstantial account of the Regimen, &c. which enabled him to bear up against them,—which forms the most valuable collection of observations on *Nervous Complaints,* that experience and liberality have yet presented to the public.

One page of PERSONAL EXPERIENCE, *is worth folios of theoretic Fancies,—or Clinical Cases,* which can only be illuminated by the twilight of conjecture: —they may be faithful narratives of the accounts given by Patients, yet, as these are very often imposed upon by their imagination attributing effects to very different causes than those which produce them, they are often very inaccurate deductions.

THE DELICATE AND THE NERVOUS, will derive the greatest advantage from keeping *a Register of their Health,*—they should note, and avoid whatever disagrees with them,—and endeavour to ascertain, what kind and quantity of Food—Exercise—Occupation and Pleasures, &c. are most agreeable to their constitution, and take them at those regular periods which appear most convenient to them. However this advice may excite the smiles of those who are swelling "in all the pride of superfluous Health," such methodical movements will considerably improve the enjoyment, and prolong the life of the Valetudinary and the Aged: for whom, Instinct is the best Guide in the choice of Aliment.

None but the most obstinately ignorant Visionary, would dream of laying down absolute Rules[86] for governing the caprice and whims of the infirm Stomachs of Crazy Valetudinarians. Codes of Dietetics[87] are almost useless,—the suggestions of Reason are often in direct opposition to the desires of Appetite.

In most matters regarding the adjustment of that supreme organ of existence,—the STOMACH,—"honest Instinct[88] comes a Volunteer."— *Ventriloquism* seldom falls to make out a fair title, to be called "unerring." A due respect to the suggestions of Instinct, every Invalid will find highly advantageous,—natural longing has frequently pointed out Food—by which *Acute Diseases* have been cured, when the most consummate medical skill was at fault, and Life at its lowest ebb.

It is needless to insist upon the importance of Diet and Regimen in *Chronic Disorders*.

Be content with ONE[89] Dish,—from want of submission to this salutary rule of Temperance—as many men dig their Grave with their *Teeth*, as with the *Tankard*;—DRUNKENNESS is deplorably destructive, but her demurer sister GLUTTONY destroys an hundred to her one.

Instinct speaks pretty plainly to those whose instruments of Digestion are in a delicate state—and is an infinitely surer guide than any Dietetic rules that can be contrived.

That the Food which we fancy most—generally sits easiest on the Stomach —is a fact which the experience of almost every individual can confirm.

The functions of Digestion go on merrily when exercised by Aliment which the Stomach asks for—they often labour in vain when we eat merely because it is the usual hour of Dining—or out of necessity, to amuse the Gastric juices, and "lull the grinding stomach's hungry rage."

To affirm that any thing is wholesome, or unwholesome,—without considering the subject in all the circumstances to which it bears relation, and the unaccountable peculiarities of different Constitutions,—is, with submission, talking nonsense.

Let every Man consult his Stomach;—to eat and drink such things—and in such quantities—as agree with that perfectly well, is wholesome for him, whilst they continue to do so[90]:—that which satisfies and refreshes us, and causes no uneasiness after, may safely be taken in moderation—whenever the Appetite is keen—whether it be at Dinner or Supper.

What we have been longest used to, is most likely to agree with us best.

The wholesomeness, &c. of all Food, depends very much on the quality of it—and the way in which it is cooked.

Those who are poor in Health, must live as they can;—certainly the less Stimulus any of us use the better, provided it be sufficient to properly carry on the Circulation:—I sometimes hold it lawful to excite Appetite when it is feeble by Age, or debilitated by Indisposition.

Those Stimuli which excite the circulation at the least expense of nervous irritation—and afford the greatest quantity of nutriment, must be most acceptable to the Stomach, when it demands restorative diet.

A healthful impetus may be given to the System by a well seasoned *Soup*, or a restorative *Ragout*, at half the expense to the machinery of Life, than by the use of those Spirituous Stimuli—which fan a feverish fire—exciting action without supplying the expenditure of the principle producing it—and merely quicken the circulation for a few minutes, without contributing any material to feed the Lamp of Life—which, if it be originally or organically defective—or is impaired by Time or Disease—will sometimes not burn brightly, unless it be supplied with the best oil, and trimmed in the most skilful manner.

Good *Mock Turtle*, see (No. 246, or 247*,) will agree with weak stomachs surprisingly well; so will that made by BIRCH *in Cornhill*, and by KAY *at Albion House*, Aldersgate Street.—This excellent Soup, is frequently ordered for Dyspeptic patients, by the senior Physician to one of the largest hospitals in this Metropolis: as a man of science and talent, certainly in as high estimation as any of his cotemporaries.

Ox-tail Soup (No. 240,) Giblet Soup (No. 244,) and (No. 87,) and (No. 89,) (No. 489,) and (No. 503,) are very agreeable extempore Restoratives,—so easy of digestion, that they are a sinecure to the Stomach, and give very little trouble to the chylopoietic organs—those whose Teeth are defective—and those whose Circulation is below *par,*—will find them acceptable Foods. "*Experto crede,*"—the reader will remember *Baglivi's* chapter "*de*

Idolis Medicorum," wherein he tells us, that "Physicians always prescribe to others, what they like themselves." The learned MANDEVILLE has favoured us with five pages on the incomparably invigorating virtues of *Stock Fish*!! a kind of Cod which is dried without being salted. See pages 316, &c. of his *Treatise on Hypochondriasis.*

The best Answers, to all inquiries about *The Wholesomes,* are the following Questions;—"Do you like it?" "Does it agree with you?"—"then eat in moderation, and you cannot do very wrong."

Those who have long lived luxuriously, to be sufficiently nourished, must be regularly supplied with Food that is nutritive, and Drink that is stimulating[91],—*Spice and Wine,* are as needful to the "BON VIVANT" of a certain Age—as its *Mother's Milk,* is to a NEW-BORN BABE.

The decrease of the energy of Life arises from the decrease of the action of the organs of the Body—especially those of Digestion,—which in early life is so intense and perfect, that a Child, after its common unexcitant meal of Bread and Milk, is as hilarious and frolicsome as an Adult person is after a certain quantity of Roast Beef and Port.

The infirm stomachs of Invalids, require a little indulgence[92]—like other bad instruments, they often want oiling, and screwing, and winding up and adjusting with the utmost care, to keep them in tolerable order;—and will receive the most salutary Stimulus, from now and then making a full meal of a favourite dish. This is not a singular notion of my own, though it may not exactly agree with the fastidious fancy of *Dr. Sangrado's* disciples,— that Starvation and Phlebotomy, are Sovereign Remedies for all Disorders.

Those philanthropic Physicians, Dr. Diet,—Dr. Quiet,—and Dr. Merryman, —hold the same doctrine as the *Magnus Coquus—i. e.* the Author of "the Cook's Oracle," to whose culinary skill we have been so repeatedly indebted in the composition of this work.

As excessive Eating and Drinking is certainly the most frequent cause of the disorders of the Rich,—so privation is the common source of complaints among the Poor;—the cause of the one, is the cure of the other —but where one of the latter dies of Want, how many thousands of the former are destroyed by Indigestion!

If strong Spices and savoury Herbs excite appetite—they (in an increased ratio,) accelerate the action of the Bowels—and hurry the food through the alimentary canal, too rapidly to allow the Absorbents to do their work properly.

Salt is the most salubrious and easily obtainable relish which Nature has given us to give sapidity to other substances; and has this advantage over all other Sauces, that if taken to excess—it carries its remedy with it in its Aperient quality.

We suspect that most mischief is done by the immoderate and constant use of the *Common Condiments.*—We have seen some puritanical folks, who are for ever boasting that *They never touch* Made Dishes, &c. (one would suppose they had the *Tongue of Pityllus*[93],) so be-devil every morsel they put into their Mouth—with Pepper, and Mustard, &c. that they made their common food ten times more *piquante*—than the burn-gullet *Bonne Bouche* of an eastern Nabob, or *a Broiled Devil*, enveloped in "veritable Sauce d'Enfer."—See (No. 355 and 538).

We do not condemn the moderate use of Spices, but the constant and excessive abuse of them,—by which the papillary nerves of the tongue become so blunted, that in a little time they lose all relish for useful nourishing food, and the Epicure is punished with all the sufferings of incessant and incurable Indigestion,—perturbed Sleep—and the horrors of the Night-Mare, &c. &c.—However, enough has been written by a thousand cautionists, to convince any rational creature of the advantage resulting to both the Body and the Mind from a simple and frugal fare:—the great secret of Health and Longevity is to keep up the sensibility of the Stomach.

No Regimen[94] can be contrived that will suit every body.

> "Try all the bounties of this fertile Globe,
> There is not such a salutary Food
> As suits with every Stomach."
>> Dr. Armstrong's *Art of Preserving Health*, book ii.
> line 120.

"I knew a black servant of Mr. Pitt, an Indian Merchant in America, who was fond of Soup *made of* Rattle Snakes,—in which the Head, without any regard to the Poison, was boiled along with the rest of the animal."—Dr. G. Fordyce, *on Digestion*, &c. 8vo. 1791, p. 119.

No food is so delicious that it pleases all palates,—nothing can be more correct than the old adage, "one man's meat is another man's poison."

It would be as difficult for a Laplander, or an earth-eating Ottomaque, to convince our good citizens that Train Oil, and gutter-mud, is a more elegant relish than their favourite Turtle—as for the former to fancy that Kay or Birch's Soup can be as agreeable as the Grease and Garbage which custom has taught them to think delicious.

> "Man differs more from Man
> Than Man from Beast."—Colman.

Celsus[95] very sensibly says, that "a healthy man, under his own government, ought not to tie himself up by strict rules,—nor to abstain from any sort of food; that he ought sometimes to fast, and sometimes to feast." *Sanis, sunt omnia Sana.*

When the Stomach sends forth eructant signals of distress, for help against Indigestion, the *Peristaltic Persuaders* (see the end of this Essay) are as agreeable and effectual assistance as can be offered; and for delicate Constitutions, and those that are impaired by Age or Intemperance, are a valuable Panacea.

They derive, and deserve this name, from the peculiar mildness of their operation[96]. One or two very gently increase the action of the principal viscera, help them to do their work a little faster,—and enable the Stomach to serve with an ejectment whatever offends it,—and move it into the Bowels.

Thus *Indigestion* is easily and speedily removed,—*Appetite* restored,—(the mouths of the absorbing vessels being cleansed) *Nutrition* is facilitated,—and *Strength* of Body, and *Energy* of Mind[97], are the happy results.

If an immediate operation be desired, take some *Tincture of Rhubarb*—as a *Pill* is the most gentle and gradually operating form for a drug—a *Tincture* in which it is as it were ready digested, is the most immediate in its action.

To Make Tincture of Rhubarb.—Steep three ounces of the best Rhubarb (pounded) and half an ounce of Carraway Seeds, (pounded) in a bottle of Brandy, for ten days. A table-spoonful in a wine-glass of hot water will generally be enough.

Compound Tincture of Senna, has been recommended, especially to those who have accustomed themselves to the use of spirituous Liquors and high living. Several similar preparations are sold under the name of *Daffy's Elixir* —or as much Epsom Salt, in half a pint of *hot* water, as experience has informed you, will produce one motion,—a Tea-spoonful (*i. e.* from one to two drachms) will generally do this—especially if it be taken in the morning, fasting, *i. e.* at least half an hour before Breakfast.

The best way of covering the taste of Salt, is to put a lump of *Sugar* and a bit of thin-cut *Lemon Peel*[98] into the hot water, for a few minutes before you stir the Salt into it,—to which you may add a few grains of grated *Ginger*.

Epsom Salt is *a very speedy laxative*, often operating within an hour,—does the business required of it with great regularity,—and is more uniform in what it does,—and when it does it,—than any Aperient;—ten minutes after you have taken it, encourage its operation by drinking half a pint, or more, of warm water—weak Broth—Tea—thin Gruel (No. 572), with some salt and butter in it—or *Soda Water* (No. 481.*) See Index.

"Nil tam ad sanitatem, et longevitatem conducit, quam crebræ et domesticæ purgationes."—Lord Bacon.—*i. e.* "Nothing contributes so much to preserve Health, and prolong Life, as frequently cleansing the alimentary canal with gentle laxatives."

We perfectly agree with Lord Bacon, and believe that in nine cases out of ten, for which Tonic Medicines are administered, *Peristaltic Persuaders* will not only much more certainly improve Appetite,—but invigorate the Constitution; by facilitating the absorption of nutriment,—which, in aged and debilitated people, is often prevented by the mouths of the vessels being half closed by the accumulation of viscid mucus, &c.

Aperient Medicine does enough, if it increases the customary Evacuation,— and does too much,—if it does more,—than excite one additional motion.

Bowels which are forced into double action to-day—must, consequently, be costive to-morrow, and Constipation will be caused by the remedy you have recourse to to remove it,—this has given rise to a *Vulgar Error,*—that the use of even the mildest Laxative is followed by Costiveness.

Rhubarb is particularly under this prejudice,—because it has been more frequently employed as a domestic remedy,—and unadvisedly administered in either too little, or too large a Dose. It has, however, been recommended by a Physician of acknowledged Ability, and extensive Experience.

"If the Bowels are constipated, they should be kept regular by a Pill of Rhubarb of five grains every morning."—PEMBERTON *on the Abdominal Viscera*, p. 113.

People are often needlessly uneasy about the Action of their Bowels.—If their general Health is good, and they have neither Head-ach nor other deranged sensations, and they live temperately, during the second period of Life, whether they have two motions in one day, or one in two days, perhaps is not of much consequence;—however, that the Alvine Exoneration should take place regularly is certainly most desirable;—especially after *Thirty-Five* years of age[99], when the elasticity of the machinery of Life begins to diminish.

To acquire a Habit of Regularity, Mr. LOCKE, who was a Physician as well as a Philosopher, advises that "if any person, as soon as he has breakfasted, would presently solicit nature, so as to obtain a stool, he might in time, by a constant application, bring it to be habitual." He says "I have known none who have been steady in the prosecution of this plan, who did not in a few months obtain the desired success."—*On Education*, p. 23, &c.

"It is well known that the alvine evacuation is periodical, and subjected to the power of habit; if the regular call is not obeyed, the necessity for the evacuation passes away; and the call being again and again neglected, habitual costiveness is the consequence."—HAMILTON *on Purgatives*, p. 72.

It will facilitate the acquirement of this salutary evacuation,—to take at night—such a dose of an Aperient medicine, as Experience has pointed out, as just sufficient to assist nature to produce a Motion in the Morning.

HABITUAL COSTIVENESS is not curable by Drugs alone,—and is most agreeably corrected by *Diet and Regimen*, those most important, and only effectual, although much neglected (because little understood) means of permanently alleviating *Chronic Complaints*, for which

"Coquina est optima Medicina."

Strong Constitutions are generally *Costive*[100],—that perfect and vigorous action of the absorbents, which is the cause of their strength, is also the cause of their Constipation:—

"Oportet sanorum, sedes esse figuratas."

This ought to make them content,—but the Constipated are for ever murmuring about a habit—which, if managed with moderate care,—is the fundamental basis of Health and Long Life. A little attention to Regimen will generally prevent it—a simple Laxative will suffice to remove it—and neither will be often necessary, for those who observe a deobstruent Diet— take proper Exercise in a pure Air—sufficient liquid Food—and eat freely of Butter, Salt, and Sugar.

The peculiarity of most Constitutions is so convenient, that almost all Costive persons—by attending to the effects which various things produce upon their Bowels—may find, in their usual Food and Drink, the means of persuading their sluggish Viscera to vibrate with healthful celerity.

A SUPPER or BREAKFAST of thin Gruel, (No. 572,) with plenty of Butter and Salt in it,—ripe Fruits, particularly *Grapes*[101],—Oranges,—Strawberries, —Raspberries,—Mulberries,—Marmalade,—Honey,—Treacle,—roasted Apples,—stewed Prunes,—Figs,—Raisins,—Tamarinds,—French Plumbs, &c.;—will almost always produce the desired effect.

Two or three strong *Cinnamon or Ginger Lozenges*, (see page 234,) gradually dissolved in the mouth when the Stomach is empty, will act as an Aperient on many persons.

SALAD OIL is a very pleasant *Peristaltic Persuader*:—by the following means it may be introduced (as a supper) to the most delicate Stomach,— without any offence to the most fastidious Palate.

Put a table-spoonful of Sherry into a wine-glass—on this a table-spoonful of Olive Oil—on this another table-spoonful of Sherry—or rub together a table-spoonful or two of Oil, with the yolk of an Egg boiled hard, (No. 547,) add a little Vinegar and Salt to it, and eat it at Supper as a Sauce to a Salad (No. 138*) of Mustard and Cresses,—or Lettuce,—Radishes,—Button Onions,—Celery,—Cucumber, &c.;—or cold boiled Asparagus,—Brocoli,—Cauliflower,—Carrot,—or Turnip,—Kidney or French Beans,—or Pease;—or Pickled Salmon, (No. 161,) Lobster, (No. 176,) Shrimps, Herrings, Sprats, (No. 170**,) or Mackarel, (No. 168,) or as a Sauce to cold Meat, &c.

You may give it an infinite variety of agreeable flavours; the ingredients to produce which are enumerated in (No. 372) of "THE COOK'S ORACLE."

Hypochondriac people are fond of taking Medicine at certain times, the spring and fall,—at the full or the new Moon, &c. whether they want it or not.—For those in Health to attempt to improve it by taking Physic, is absurd indeed. Remember the epitaph on the Italian Count—

> "I was well—
> Wished to be better—
> Took Physic—and died."

Hypochondriasis—Spleen—Vapours—the Blue Devils—the Bile—Nervous Debility, &c. are but so many different names for those Disorders which arise either from CHRONIC WEAKNESS of the Constitution—or an inconsiderate management of it.—A man who has a strong stamina will bear irregularities with impunity—which will soon destroy a more delicate frame.

We do not laugh at the melancholy of the Hypochondriac,—or consider his Complaints as merely the hallucinations of *un Malade Imaginaire*; but trace the cause of them to either some Indigestion interrupting the functions of the Alimentary Canal—which a gentle Aperient would immediately remove—or the ineffective performance of the Restorative Process—insufficiently nutritive Diet—or depression of the vital and animal functions from anxiety or over-exertion of either the Mind or the Body:—which nothing but Rest and nutritive Food can repair.

The Editor of this little treatise has had from his Youth to bear up against an highly irritable nervous system,—the means he has found useful to manage and support it, he is now recording for the benefit of other Nervous Invalids.

We advise our Friends—never to call in even the gentle aid of Peristaltic Persuaders,—but when Instinct absolutely insists upon it—some of the Indications of which are, "A disagreeable taste in the Mouth—Eructations —Want of Appetite—Sensations of distention in the Stomach and Bowels —Pains in the Stomach or Head—Vertigo—Feverishness—Restlessness— Peevishness," &c.—but these will often disappear by taking a liquid meal, instead of a solid one, or using more exercise, will often answer the purpose.—Mr. Jones very sensibly observes, "if people will by no means rest from constantly tampering with laxatives, instead of using exercise, the habit of using the *Lavement* every evening cannot be so destructive, as it irritates only *twelve inches* of intestine, and spares raking down the other *thirty-nine feet.*"—*See Med. Vul. Errors,* p. 44.

RELAXED BOWELS[102] are often extremely unmanageable, and difficult to regulate—and are the principal cause of that *Chronic Weakness* which is so generally complained of, and of many other distressing Nervous Disorders.

If the Bowels are unfaithful to the Stomach, and, instead of playing fair,— let go their hold of the "Pabulum Vitæ," before the Absorbents have properly performed the process which that grand organ has prepared for them—Nutrition will be deficient; and Flatulence, &c. &c. Giddiness,— Spasms,—Head-ache,—and Back-ache,—and what are called *Bilious and Nervous* Disorders,—and all the Diseases incident to Debility, will attack you on the slightest cause.

Those who are afflicted with a relaxation of the Bowels, are advised to a *Dry diet,* rather than a *Liquid one,* and must submit to a Regimen diametrically contrary to that we have recommended to cure Constipation.

"Since I lessened my Drink I have been much more costive than I was before, and have for two years past freed myself from a Diarrhœa. Costiveness generally attends dry food in other animals as well as men."— B. ROBINSON, *on Food and Discharges,* p. 82 and 64.

Live principally upon Animal Food sufficiently cooked, and Stale Bread, or biscuit;—instead of Malt liquor (unless it be very mild and good Homebrewed Beer, which is the best of all Beverages) drink Beef-Tea, (No. 563), or well made Toast and Water[103] (No. 463*), with about one-fourth part of Wine, and a little Sugar and grated Nutmeg or Ginger in it;—if the Stomach be troubled with Acidity, or great Flatulence, one-eighth part of Brandy may agree with it better:—*whatever You eat and drink should be Warmed.*—See page 94 on *Siesta,* and page 158.

Be watchful of the effects of the Food which you take,—avoid whatever appears to irritate, and *eat only that which experience has proved acceptable.*

IRRITABLE BOWELS are excited to inconveniently increased action by any thing that the Stomach has either not the ability, or the inclination, to prepare for them,—and *Diarrhœa* is the consequence.

The easiest and most effectual method of restoring tranquillity in the Bowels—is to be content with a light diet of Gruel, Broth, or Fish, &c. till the return of a keen Appetite assures you, that the Stomach has recovered its powers, and being ready for action, requires its usual supply of solid food.

When the Bowels get a trick of emptying themselves too often,—a teaspoonful of Compound Powder of Chalk in your Tea,—or a wine-glassful of the following mixture, taken twice or thrice a day, will generally cure them of it very speedily:—

> ℞ Chalk mixture, six ounces.
> Tincture of Cinnamon (No. 416*), one ditto.
> Opiate Confection, one drachm.
> Mixed together.

If Diarrhœa continues obstinate, more powerful Astringents[104] may be necessary.

TINCTURE OF CINNAMON (No. 416*) is one of the best cordial tonics—see also (No. 569) and (Nos. 413 & 15.)

OPIUM LOZENGES, containing a quarter of a grain each, and strongly flavoured with Oil of Peppermint, are recommended to those who are troubled with relaxed Bowels.

STRONG PEPPERMINT LOZENGES are the most convenient portable carminative:
—as soon as they are dissolved, their influence is felt from the beginning, to
the end of the Alimentary Canal;—they dissipate flatulence so immediately,
that they well deserve the name of *Vegetable Æther*; and are recommended
to SINGERS[105] AND PUBLIC SPEAKERS, as giving effective excitement to the
organs of the Voice,—as a support against the distressing effects of fasting
too long—and to give energy to the Stomach between meals.

N.B. *Sixty different sorts of Lozenges*, are made in the most superlative
manner, by Mr. Smith, Fell Street, Wood Street, Cheapside.

His *Rose Jujubes*—are a very elegant preparation, which those who have
not a remarkably Sweet Breath, are recommended to take the last thing at
night, and the first in the morning—the breath smells faintest when the
Stomach is emptiest.

His *Mellifluous Aromatics* are so delicately flavoured, they moisten the
mouth and throat without cloying the Palate, Stomach, &c., which is more
than can be said of most Lozenges.

To make FORTY PERISTALTIC PERSUADERS.

> Take,
>> Turkey Rhubarb, finely pulverized, two drachms.
>> Syrup (by weight) one drachm.
>> Oil of Carraway, ten drops (minums).
> Made into Pills, each of which will contain *Three Grains of Rhubarb*.

THE DOSE OF THE PERSUADERS must be adapted to the constitutional
peculiarity of the Patient:—when you wish to accelerate or augment the
Alvine Exoneration—take two, three, or more, according to the effect you
desire to produce—*two Pills* will do as much for one person as *five* or *six*
will for another; they generally will very regularly perform what you wish
to-day,—without interfering with what you hope will happen to-morrow;—
and are, therefore, as convenient an argument against Constipation as any
we are acquainted with.

The most convenient opportunity to introduce them to the Stomach—is early
in the Morning, when it is unoccupied,—and has no particular business to

attend to, *i. e.* at least half an hour before Breakfast.

Physic should never interrupt the Stomach, when it is engaged in digesting *Food*—perhaps the best time to take it, is when you awake out of your first Sleep—or as soon as you awake in the morning. Moreover, such is the increased sensibility of some Stomachs at that time, that half the quantity of Medicine will suffice.

From *two to four Persuaders* will generally produce one additional motion within twelve hours.

They may be taken at any time—by the most DELICATE FEMALES, whose Constitutions are so often distressed by Constipation[106], and destroyed by the drastic purgatives they take to relieve it. See also page 224.

Their agreeable flavour recommends them as the most convenient aperient for CHILDREN, whose indispositions most frequently arise from obstructions in the Bowels;—it is not always a very easy task to prevail upon a spoiled Child to take Physic;—therefore—we have made our Pill to taste exactly like Gingerbread.

For INFANTS, too young to swallow a Pill, pound it, and mix it with Currant Jelly, Honey, or Treacle.

ON THE FIRST ATTACK OF DISEASE—it may generally be disarmed by discharging the contents of the Bowels:—IN EVERY DISORDER[107] the main point is carefully to watch, and constantly to keep up the activity of the Alimentary Canal—for want of due attention to this, MILLIONS (especially of *Children*) HAVE DIED OF MEDICABLE DISORDERS!!

FOR BILIOUS OR LIVER[108] COMPLAINTS, (which are now the fashionable names for all those deranged sensations of the Abdominal Viscera—which as often arise from the want, as from the excess of Bile—and perhaps most frequently from *Indigestion*)—and for expelling WORMS[109], for which it is the fashion to administer *Mercury*[110] (which, because it is the only remedy for one Disease, people suppose must be a *panacea* for every disorder) and other drastic mineral medicines, which are awfully uncertain both in their strength and in their operation.

If, instead of two or three times a week tormenting your Bowels with *Corrosive Cathartics,—Hydragogues,—Phlegmagogues,* &c., you take one or two gentle PERSUADERS, twice or thrice a day;—they will excite a gradual and regularly increased action of the Viscera—restore the tone of the Alimentary tube—and speedily and effectually cure the disorder, without injuring the Constitution.

There is not a more universal or more mischievous *Vulgar Error*, than the notion, that Physic is efficacious, in proportion as it is extremely disagreeable to take, and frightfully violent in its operation,—unless a medicine actually produces more Distress in the System, than the Disorder it is administered to remove—in fact, if the Remedy be not worse than the Disease, the million have no faith in it—and are not satisfied that they can be perfectly cured if they escape Phlebotomy,—unless put to extreme pain, and plentifully supplied with Black Doses, and drastic Drugs;—they have the best opinion of that Doctor who most furiously

"Vomits—Purges—Blisters—Bleeds, and *Sweats 'em."*

To perfectly content them that you have most profoundly considered their case, you must to such Prescription—add a Proscription of every thing they appear particularly partial to!!!

People who in all other respects appear to be very rational—and are apt to try other questions by the rules of Common Sense, in matters relating to their Health, surrender their understanding to the fashion of the Day,—and in the present Century, on all occasions take *Calomel* as coolly as in the last, their Grandfathers inundated their poor Stomachs with *Tar-Water*.

———

TONIC TINCTURE, (No. 569) is

Peruvian Bark, bruised, one ounce and a half.
Orange Peel, do. one ounce.
Brandy, or Proof Spirit, one pint.

Let these ingredients steep for ten days, shaking the bottle every day—let it remain quiet two days—and then decant the clear liquor.

Dose—one teaspoonful in a wineglass of water, twice a day, when you feel languid, *i. e.* when the Stomach is empty, about an hour before Dinner, and in the Evening. Twenty grains of the Powder of Bark may be added to it occasionally.

To this agreeable Aromatic Tonic we are under personal obligations, for frequently putting our Stomach into good temper, and procuring us good Appetite and good Digestion.

In low Nervous affections, arising from a languid Circulation—and, when the Stomach is in a state of shabby debility from age—intemperance, or other causes—this is a most acceptable restorative.

N.B. Tea made with dried and bruised *Seville Orange Peel*, (in the same manner as common Tea,) and drank with milk and sugar, has been taken for Breakfast by *Nervous* and *Dyspeptic* persons with great benefit.

Chewing a bit of *Orange Peel* twice a day when the Stomach is empty, will be found very grateful, and strengthening to it.—

Stomachic Tinctures.

Two ounces of Cascarilla Bark (bruised)—or dried Orange Peel,—or Colomba Root—infused for a fortnight in a pint of Brandy, will give you the Tinctures called by those names.

Dose—one or two teaspoonsful in a wine-glass of water.

Tincture of Cinnamon, (No. 416*).

This excellent Cordial is made by pouring a bottle of genuine Cogniac (No. 471) on three ounces of bruised Cinnamon (Cassia will not do). This cordial restorative was more in vogue formerly, than it is now;—a teaspoonful of it, and a lump of Sugar, in a glass of good Sherry or Madeira, with the yolk of an Egg beat up in it—was called "*Balsamum Vitæ.*"

> "*Cur moriatur homo, qui sumit de Cinnamomo?*"—"Cinnamon is verie comfortable to the Stomacke, and the principall partes of the bodie."

"Ventriculum, Jecur, Lienem Cerebrum, nervosque juvant et roborat."—"I reckon it a great treasure for a student to have by him, in his closet, to take now and then a spoonfull."—COGAN'S *Haven of Health*, 4to. 1584, p. 111.

Obs.—Two teaspoonsful in a wineglass of water—are a present and pleasant remedy in Nervous Languors—and in relaxations of the Bowels—in the latter case five drops of Laudanum may be added to each dose.

SODA WATER, (No. 481*.)

The best way of producing agreeable *Pneumatic Punch,* as a learned Chemist has called this refreshing refrigerant, is to fill two half-pint Tumblers half full of Water,—stir into one 30 grains of *Carbonate of Potash,*—into the other 25 grains of *Citric[111] Acid,* (both being previously finely pounded,)—when the powders are perfectly dissolved—pour the contents of one tumbler into the other—and sparkling Soda Water is instantaneously produced.

To make DOUBLE SODA WATER, use double the quantity of the Powder.

Single Soda Water is a delightful drink in sultry weather—and may be very agreeably flavoured by dissolving a little Raspberry or Red Currant Jelly in the Water, (before you add the Carbonate of Potash to it), or a little Tincture of Ginger, (No. 411,)—or Syrup of Ginger, (No. 394,)—or Syrup of Lemon Peel, (No. 393,)—or infuse a roll of fresh and thin-cut Lemon Peel, and a bit of Sugar in the water—or rub down a few drops of (No. 408,) with a bit of Lump Sugar, with or without a little grated Ginger;—a glass of Sherry or a tablespoonful of Brandy is sometimes added.

The addition of a teaspoonful of the TONIC TINCTURE (No. 569,) will give you a very refreshing Stomachic—and ten drops of *Tinct. Ferri Muriati* put into the water in which you dissolve the Citric Acid—a fine effervescing Chalybeate.

The day after a Feast, if you feel fevered and heated, you cannot do better than drink a half-pint glass or two of *Single Soda Water* between Breakfast and Dinner.

DOUBLE SODA WATER (especially if made with tepid water) is an excellent auxiliary to accelerate the operation of Aperient Medicine—and, if taken in the Morning fasting, will sometimes move the Bowels without further assistance.

If some good *Cogniac* or Essence of Ginger (No. 411) be added to it, it is one of the best helps to set the Stomach to work—and remove the distressing languor which sometimes follows hard drinking.

ESSENCE OF GINGER, (No. 411).

The fragrant *aroma* of Ginger is so extremely volatile, that it evaporates almost as soon as it is pounded—the fine Lemon peel *goût* flies off presently.

If Ginger is taken to produce an immediate effect—to warm the Stomach—dispel Flatulence, &c., or as an addition to Aperient Medicine—the following is the best preparation of it:—

Steep three ounces of *fresh grated* Ginger, and one ounce of fresh Lemon Peel, (cut thin) in a quart of Brandy—or Proof Spirit, for ten days, shaking it up each day.

N.B. TINCTURE OF ALLSPICE, which is sometimes called *Essence of Bishop*, for making *Mulled Wine, &c.* extempore, is prepared in the same manner.

GRUEL, (No. 252).

1st. Ask those who are to eat it, if they like it *THICK* or *thin*; if the latter, mix well together by degrees, in a pint basin, *one* tablespoonful of Oatmeal with three of cold water;—if the former, *two* spoonsful.

Have ready, in a Stewpan, a pint of boiling water or milk—pour this by degrees to the Oatmeal you have mixed—return it into the Stewpan—set it on the fire—and let it boil for five minutes—stirring it all the time to prevent the Oatmeal from burning at the bottom of the Stewpan—skim—and strain it through a Hair Sieve.

2d. To convert this into CAUDLE—add a little Ale—Wine—or Brandy—with Sugar—and *if the Bowels are disordered,* a little Nutmeg or Ginger grated.

Gruel may be made with Broth[112] (No. 490,) or (No. 252,) or (No. 564,) instead of Water—(to make *Crowdie*, see No. 205*,)—and may be flavoured with *Sweet Herbs—Soup Roots* and *Savoury Spices*—by boiling them for a few minutes in the water you are going to make the Gruel with—or ZEST (No. 255)—Pea Powder (No. 458)—or dried Mint—Mushroom Catsup (No. 439)—or a few grains of Curry Powder (No. 455)—or Savoury Ragout Powder (No. 457)—or Cayenne (No. 404)—or Celery Seed bruised—or Soup Herb Powder (No. 459)—or an Onion minced very fine and bruised in with the Oatmeal—or a little Eschalot Wine (No. 402)—or Essence of Celery (No. 409)—or (No. 413)—(No. 417)—or (No. 420),&c.

PLAIN GRUEL, such as is directed in the first part of this Recipe, is one of the best Breakfasts and Suppers that we can recommend to the rational Epicure;—is the most comforting soother of an irritable Stomach that we know—and particularly acceptable to it *after a hard day's work of Intemperate Feasting*—when the addition of half an ounce of Butter, and a teaspoonful of Epsom Salt will give it an aperient quality, which will assist the principal Viscera to get rid of their burden.

"*Water Gruel*" (says Tryon in his Obs. on Health, 16mo. 1688, p. 42,) is "the KING *of Spoon Meats*," and "the QUEEN *of Soups*," and gratifies nature beyond all others.

In the "*Art of Thriving*," 1697, p. 8, are directions for preparing Fourscore Noble and Wholesome Dishes, upon most of which *a Man may live excellent well for Twopence a day*: the author's *Obs.* on *Water Gruel* is, that "ESSENCE OF OATMEAL" makes "*a noble and exhilarating meal!*"

Dr. FRANKLIN'S favourite Breakfast was a good basin of warm Gruel, in which there was a small slice of Butter with Toasted Bread and Nutmeg—the expense of this, he reckoned at three half-pence.

"Mastication is a very necessary Preparation of solid Aliment, without which there can be no good Digestion."—The above are the first lines in ARBUTHNOT'S *Essay on Aliment*.

This first act of the important process of Digestion, is most perfectly performed, when the flavour, &c. of our Food is agreeable to our Taste;—we naturally detain upon our Palate those things which please it,—and the Meat we relish most, is consequently most broken down by chewing, and most intimately incorporated with the Saliva—this is the reason why what we desire most, we digest best.

Here, is a sufficient answer, to the Folios which have sprung from the Pens of cynical and senseless Scribblers—on whom Nature not having bestowed a Palate, they have proscribed those pleasures they had not Sense[113] to taste, or comprehend the wise purposes for which they were given to us, and

> "Compound for Sins they are inclin'd to,
> By damning those they have no mind to."

How large a share of the business of Digestion is managed by Mastication, has been shown by the experiments of *Spallanzani*[114].

To Chew long, and leisurely, is the only way to extract the essence of our food—to enjoy the taste of it, and to render it easily convertible into laudable Chyle, by the facility it gives to the gastric juices to dissolve it without trouble.

The pleasure of the *Palate*, and the health of the *Stomach*, are equally promoted by this salutary habit, which all should be taught to acquire in their infancy.

The more tender meat is, the more we may eat of it.—That which is most difficult to Chew, is of course most difficult to Digest.

From 30 to 40 (according to the tenderness of the meat) has been calculated as the mean number of Munches, that solid meat requires, to prepare it for its journey down *the Red Lane*; less will be sufficient for tender, delicate, and easily digestible white meats.

The sagacious *Gourmand*, will calculate this precisely,—and not waste his precious moments in useless Jaw-work, or invite an Indigestion by neglecting *Mastication*.

I cannot give any positive rules for this, it depends on the state of the Teeth[115]; every one, especially *the Dyspeptic*, ought to ascertain the condition of these useful working tools; and to use them with proportionate diligence, is an indispensable exercise which every rational Epicure will most cheerfully perform, who has any regard for the welfare of his Stomach[116].

It has been recommended, that those whose Teeth are defective, should mince their meat—this will certainly save trouble to both Teeth and Stomach—nevertheless, it is advisable, let the meat be minced ever so fine, to endeavour to mumble it into a pulp before it be introduced to the Stomach—on account of the advantage derived from its admixture with the SALIVA.

"By experiment, I determined the quantity of *Saliva* secreted in half an hour, to be *whilst the parts were at rest*, four drachms,—whilst *eating*, five ounces four drachms."—STARK *on Diet*, p. 99.

MASTICATION is the source of all good Digestion;—*with its assistance*, almost any thing may be put into any stomach with impunity:—*without it*, Digestion is always difficult, and often impossible: and be it always remembered, it is not merely what we eat, but what we digest well, that nourishes us.

The sagacious *Gourmand* is ever mindful of his motto—

"Masticate, Denticate, Chump, Grind, and Swallow."

The four first acts, he knows he must perform properly,—before he dare attempt the fifth.

Those who cannot enjoy a savoury morsel on account of their Teeth, or rather on account of the want of them, we refer to the note at the foot of p. 260, and also have the pleasure to inform them, that PATENT MASTICATORS are made by PALMER, *Cutler, in St. James's Street.*

To those who may inadvertently exercise their Masticative faculties on unworthy materials—or longer on worthy ones than nature finds convenient, we recommend "Peristaltic Persuaders." See page 235.

When either the *Teeth* or *Stomach* are extremely feeble, especial care must be taken *to keep Meat till it is tender*—before it is cooked—and call in the aid of the *Pestle* and *Mortar*.—And see Nos. 10,—18,—87,—89,—175,—178; from 185 to 250,—502—542—and especially 503. Or dress in the usual way whatever is best liked—mince it—put it into a Mortar—and pound it with a little Broth or melted Butter,—Vegetable,—Herb,—Spice,—Zest, No. 255, &c.—according to the taste, &c. of the Eater.—The business of the Stomach is thus very materially facilitated.

"Mincing or Pounding Meat—saveth the grinding of the Teeth; and therefore (no doubt) is more nourishing, especially in Age,—or to them that have weak teeth; but Butter is not proper for weak bodies,—and therefore, moisten it in pounding with a little Claret Wine, and a very little Cinnamon or Nutmeg."—LORD BACON's *Natural History*, Century 1.—54.

This is important Advice for those who are afflicted with *"Tic Douloureux,"*—the paroxysm of which is generally provoked by the exercise of Eating,—and the Editor has known that dreadful disorder cured by the Patient frequently taking food thus prepared in small portions, instead of a regular meal.

The TEETH should be cleaned after every meal with a "TOOTH PRESERVER," (*i. e.* a very soft brush,) and then rinsed with *tepid* water—*never neglect this at night*;—nothing destroys the Teeth so fast as suffering food to stick between them—those who observe this rule, will seldom have any occasion for *Dentifrices—Essences of Ivory—Indurating Liquid Enamels, &c.*

But it is the rage just now with some Dentists, to recommend Brushes so hard, that they fetch Blood like a Lancet wherever they touch; and instead of *"Teeth Preservers,"* these should rather be termed *"Gum Bleeders."*

Not even a Philosopher can endure the TOOTHACH patiently—what an overcoming agony then it must be to a *Grand Gourmand!*—depriving him of the means of enjoying an amusement which to him is the grand solace for all sublunary cares.—To alleviate, and indeed generally to cure this intolerable pain—we recommend

Toothache and Anti-rheumatic Embrocation, (No. 567.)

> Sal Volatile—three parts.
> Laudanum—one part.

Mix and rub the part in pain therewith frequently. If the Tooth which aches is hollow, drop some of this on a bit of cotton, and put it into the Tooth,—if the pain does not abate within an hour—take out the cotton, and put another piece in—changing it every hour four or five times, till the pain ceases.

In a general Face-ach, or sore Throat—moisten a piece of flannel with it and put it to the part affected,—rub any part afflicted with Rheumatism night and morning, and in the middle of the day. I have frequently cured old and inveterate Rheumatic affections with this Liniment.

www.ingramcontent.com/pod-product-compliance
Lightning Source LLC
Chambersburg PA
CBHW080524030426
42337CB00023B/4618